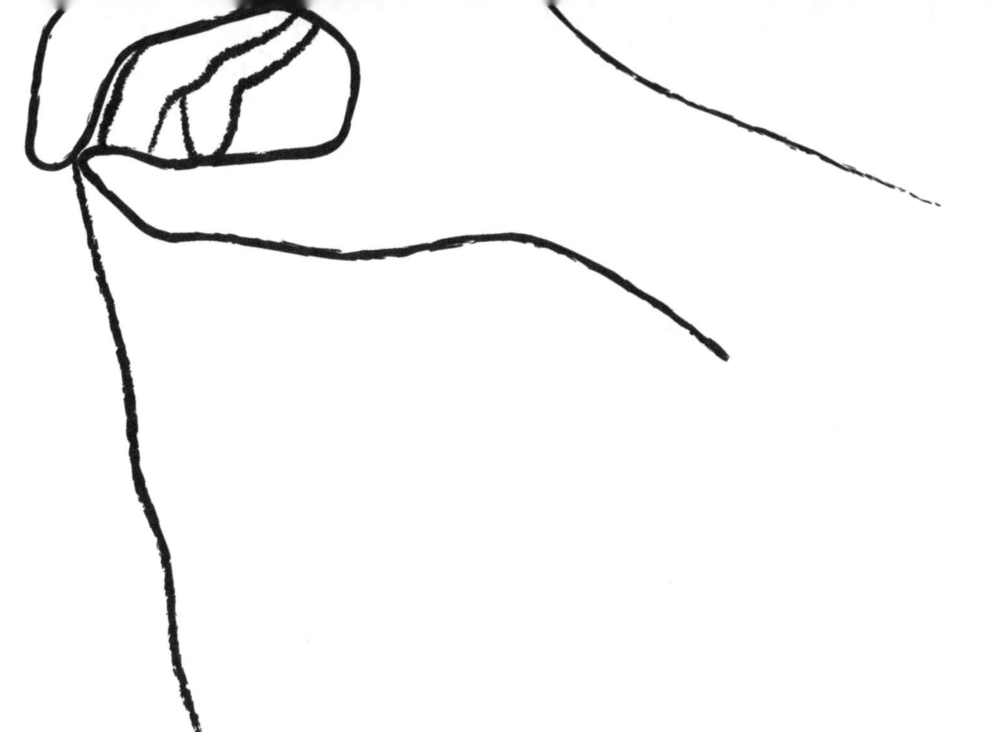

Disorganized *Attachment*
Workbook

Mending Emotional Scars, Fostering Resilience, and Nurturing Secure Relationships

Isabella Cruz

"The greatest thing you'll ever learn is just to love and be loved in return." — Eden Ahbez

Copyright **2024 Isabella Cruz**

This book is a work of non-fiction and is based on the research and experiences of the author. Some individuals' names and personal details have been changed to protect their privacy.

Acknowledgement

I am deeply grateful to Dr. Read Stevenson, for his invaluable guidance.

My heartfelt appreciation to Dr. Jenny White, for her unwavering encouragement.

I acknowledge the immense contributions of Joel and Craig.

Finally, my deepest gratitude goes to David and Bella, for their unwavering love and support.

About the Author

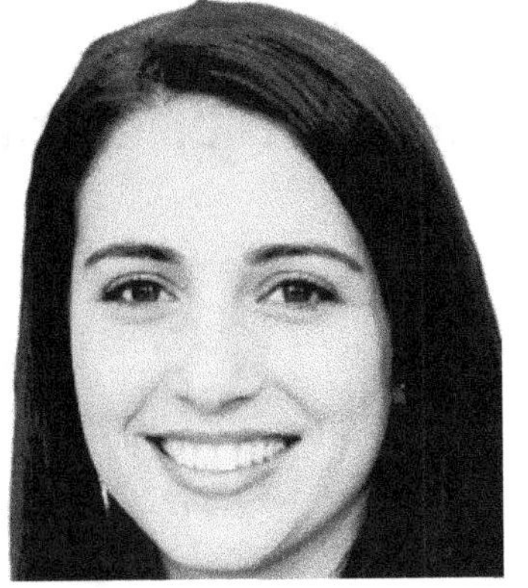

Isabella Cruz is a renowned psychologist and resilience coach, known for her empowering and relatable approach to mental health. Holding a doctorate in Psychology from Stanford University, she specializes in cognitive-behavioral therapy and mindfulness techniques.

With extensive experience in clinical practice, Isabella has dedicated her career to helping individuals overcome mental barriers and achieve emotional freedom. She lives in Seattle, where she continues to inspire and support others through her practice, coaching, and public speaking.

Other Books by this same author includes:

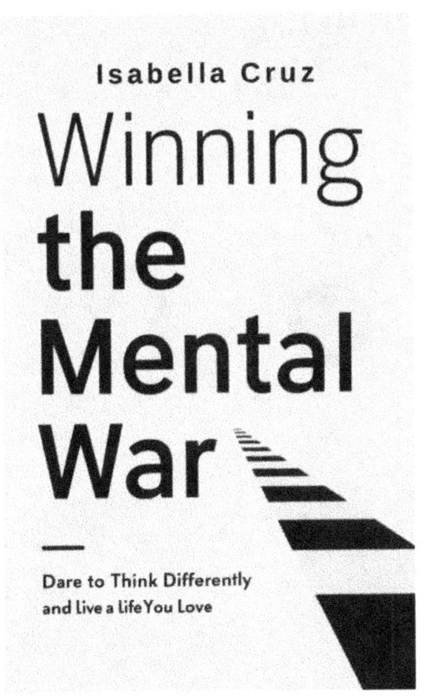

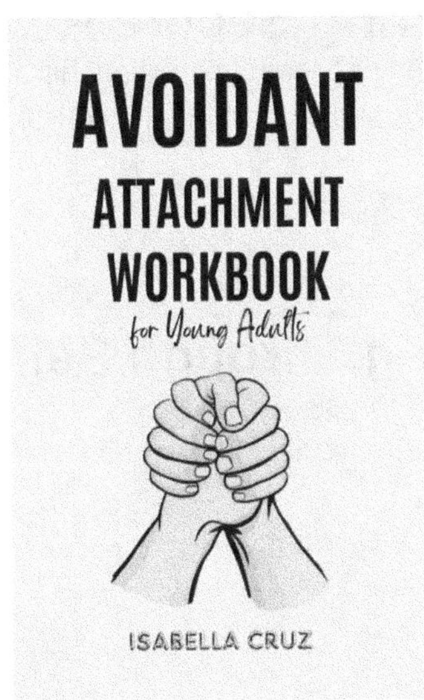

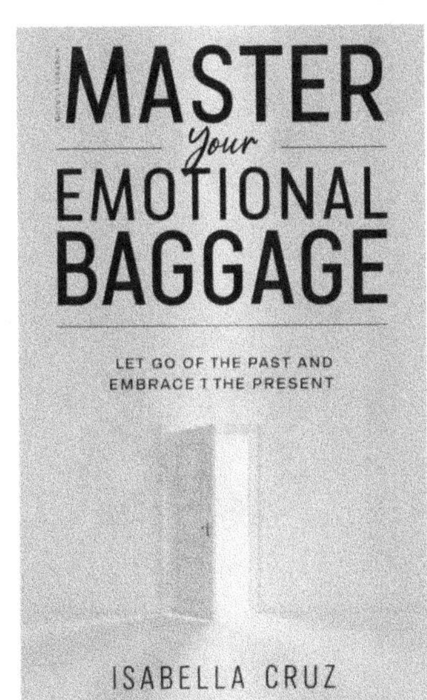

Table
Of Contents

How To Use This Workbook

Start with Self-Reflection: Begin by setting aside some quiet time to reflect on your personal experiences with attachment. This will help you connect with the material on a deeper level.

Read Each Chapter Carefully: Work through each chapter at your own pace. Take your time to understand the concepts and how they apply to your life.

Complete the Exercises: After reading, engage with the exercises provided. They are designed to help you explore your thoughts, emotions, and behaviors related to avoidant attachment.

Journal Your Thoughts: Use the space provided to jot down your thoughts, insights, and any patterns you notice as you work through the exercises.

Practice Consistently: Consistency is key. Set aside regular time each week to work on the exercises, even if it's just a few minutes a day.

Reflect and Review: Periodically, go back and review your notes and completed exercises. Reflect on your progress and how your understanding of avoidant attachment has evolved.

Apply What You Learn: Begin to apply the insights and strategies you've gained in your daily life. Notice how your relationships and interactions change as you grow.

Revisit as Needed: This workbook is a tool for ongoing growth. Feel free to revisit sections as your understanding deepens or as new challenges arise.

"We are born in relationship, we are wounded in relationship, and we can be healed in relationship." — Harville Hendrix

Introduction

James walked into my office on a rainy Tuesday afternoon, his posture stiff, his eyes darting nervously around the room. He was in his late thirties, dressed in a crisp suit that looked freshly pressed, but his hands trembled slightly as he handed me the intake form.

From the outside, James seemed like someone who had it all—a successful career as a financial analyst in downtown Seattle, a beautiful home, and a family that appeared picture-perfect. Yet, as we sat down to talk, it became clear that something was deeply troubling him.

James had come to me for help with anxiety, which he said had been plaguing him for years. He described how he would lie awake at night, heart pounding, convinced that something terrible was going to happen.

During the day, he found himself overreacting to small things, snapping at his colleagues or withdrawing from his wife and children.

Despite his outward success, James confessed that he felt like an imposter, always on the verge of losing everything he had worked so hard to achieve.

As we dug deeper into his history, James began to reveal a childhood that was anything but stable. He had grown up in foster care, shuffled from one home to another, never staying long enough to form lasting bonds.

His biological parents had been absent, caught in a cycle of addiction and neglect, leaving James to fend for himself from a young age. The constant upheaval left him with a pervasive sense of insecurity, and he had learned early on that the only person he could rely on was himself.

It wasn't long before I began to see the pattern of disorganized attachment emerging. James had developed a deep-seated fear of abandonment, which manifested as anxiety and a need for control.

His relationships, both personal and professional, were marked by a push-pull dynamic—he desperately craved connection, yet he feared it would be taken away from him at any moment.

This fear drove him to sabotage his closest relationships, pushing people away just when they got too close, convinced that it was only a matter of time before they left him anyway.

But what stood out most about James was the profound self-sabotage he engaged in. As we worked together, it became clear that his greatest fear wasn't just that others would abandon him—it was that he would never be able to escape the cycle of fear and insecurity that had defined his life.

He had internalized the belief that he was fundamentally unworthy of love and stability, and this belief fueled his anxiety and self-destructive behaviors.

Our sessions were challenging. There were moments when James would retreat, shutting down emotionally, or lash out in frustration when we touched on particularly painful memories.

But there were also moments of breakthrough, where he began to see the connections between his past and his present.

He started to recognize the patterns that had been playing out in his life for decades—the way he would push his wife away whenever they began to get close, or how he would overextend himself at work to prove his worth, only to burn out and withdraw.

The turning point came when James, after months of therapy, finally admitted that his greatest fear was not that others would abandon him, but that he would abandon himself. He feared that no matter how much he tried to heal, he would always be trapped in the same cycle of fear and self-doubt.

Disorganized attachment is a complex and often misunderstood attachment style that typically develops in childhood as a result of inconsistent, frightening, or chaotic caregiving.

Children with disorganized attachment often experience their caregivers as both a source of comfort and a source of fear, leading to confusion and insecurity. This attachment style can manifest in adulthood as a pervasive sense of mistrust, difficulty in forming healthy relationships, and a tendency to engage in self-sabotaging behaviors.

Individuals with disorganized attachment may find themselves caught in a cycle of seeking closeness and then pushing it away, fearing both intimacy and abandonment.

This can lead to significant challenges in both personal and professional relationships, as well as ongoing struggles with self-worth and emotional regulation.

Understanding your attachment style is the first step towards creating healthier, more secure relationships and a more resilient sense of self.

Do You Have a Disorganized Attachment Style?

Answer "Yes" or "No" to the following questions:

Do you often feel conflicted about wanting closeness in relationships but then feel anxious or uncomfortable when you get it?

- *Yes*
- *No*

Have you ever found yourself pushing someone away because you feared they would eventually leave you?
- *Yes*
- *No*

Do you struggle to trust others, even when there's no clear reason to doubt them?
- *Yes*
- *No*

Do you frequently worry that something will go wrong in your relationships, even when things seem fine?
- *Yes*
- *No*

Is it difficult for you to express your emotions or needs in relationships because you fear rejection or abandonment?
- *Yes*
- *No*

Did you experience significant instability or inconsistency in your relationships during childhood?
- *Yes*
- *No*

Do you tend to switch between idealizing and devaluing the people you care about?

- *Yes*
- *No*

Have you noticed that your relationships often feel chaotic or unpredictable?

- *Yes*
- *No*

Do you have a pattern of self-sabotaging your relationships, like creating conflict or distancing yourself when things get too close?

- *Yes*
- *No*

Do you frequently feel like you have to be on guard or "walk on eggshells" in your relationships to avoid conflict or rejection?

- *Yes*
- *No*

Scoring:

- *If you answered "Yes" to five or more questions, you may have a disorganized attachment style.*
- *If you answered "Yes" to fewer than five questions, you might not have a disorganized attachment style, but it's still worth exploring any patterns you notice.*

Chapter 1

UNDERSTANDING DISORGANIZED ATTACHMENT

I hadn't seen Laura in years when I unexpectedly ran into her at a psychology conference in Seattle. The city had changed so much since we'd last met, with new skyscrapers casting shadows over the old familiar streets. I spotted her across the crowded room, and the recognition was instant. She hadn't changed much—still radiating that vibrant energy that made her so magnetic. We exchanged warm hugs and started catching up over coffee.

Laura had become a successful lawyer, a testament to her resilience. Yet, as we talked, I noticed a shadow of detachment in her eyes, a hint of something unresolved.

She mentioned her recent discovery of a half-sister she had never known existed.

Her mother, who had remarried after Laura's father passed away, had had another child—a girl who had been raised in a stable, loving environment, far from the chaos of Laura's childhood.

Laura had met her sister only a few months earlier and had been grappling with complex feelings ever since. This sister had a life that Laura had longed for—one marked by stability, love, and continuity.

The twist in Laura's story was that, instead of feeling joy for her sister, she experienced an overwhelming mix of resentment and envy. It was as though the discovery had opened up old wounds rather than healed them.

Laura's struggle with these emotions came to a head during a family gathering where her sister was present. In a moment of vulnerability, Laura revealed to me that she had acted out of character, creating a scene that led to a fallout with her sister.

This was the first time Laura had truly confronted the depth of her unresolved attachment issues.

She was torn between the longing for the stable upbringing her sister had received and the harsh reality of her own turbulent past.

Seeing Laura navigate this emotional turmoil was both poignant and eye-opening. It underscored how disorganized attachment patterns don't just affect romantic relationships but can reverberate throughout all aspects of one's life.

Laura's reaction to meeting her sister illustrated how deeply ingrained her childhood experiences had become, influencing her sense of self and her capacity for trust and connection.

Pamela C. Regan's insight highlights a crucial aspect of human development: our initial relationships with our parents shape our sense of self. These early interactions can lay the groundwork for either security and trust or confusion and fear.

For some, these formative experiences build a foundation of trust that supports healthy relationships throughout life.

For others, the experience is more complicated, marked by uncertainty and a deep yearning for connection. This complexity is characteristic of disorganized attachment, an attachment style that affects a significant number of people and is often misunderstood.

If you are working through this workbook, you might be dealing with the impacts of disorganized attachment. You may find yourself struggling with overwhelming emotions, difficulty in trusting others, or a persistent sense of inner conflict.

You might experience a push-pull dynamic in relationships, where you both desire closeness and fear intimacy. These feelings are common among those with disorganized attachment, and you are not alone in navigating this path.

Disorganized attachment arises from caregiving environments that were inconsistent, frightening, or both. As infants and young children, we depend on caregivers to offer safety, comfort, and emotional regulation.

When caregivers are overwhelmed, fearful, or abusive, the messages we receive become mixed.

We learn to link love with fear and safety with danger, leading to a deep internal conflict that can affect us throughout our lives.

Imagine a child seeking comfort from a parent only to be met with anger or indifference. Or a parent who is intermittently loving and attentive but also becomes distant or frightening.

These experiences create a sense of unpredictability and chaos, leaving the child feeling confused and insecure. The child's brain, unable to reconcile these conflicting messages, develops a disorganized attachment style as a coping mechanism.

The impact of disorganized attachment can be extensive. It can influence our ability to form healthy relationships, regulate emotions, and trust ourselves and others. We might struggle with anxiety, depression, low self-esteem, and a heightened sensitivity to rejection.

We may find ourselves attracted to unhealthy relationships or repeatedly falling into painful patterns from the past.

Despite these challenges, disorganized attachment is not a permanent condition. With understanding, support, and deliberate effort, you can heal from past wounds and work toward improved emotional well-being.

This workbook is designed to support you on this journey, providing tools and insights to help you understand your attachment style, develop coping strategies, and build healthier relationships.

CHARACTERISTICS AND ORIGINS

Disorganized attachment isn't just a simple label; it represents a complex set of behaviors and internal experiences shaped by inconsistent, frightening, or neglectful caregiving.

It's a survival mechanism developed in response to early childhood challenges.

When a child's primary caregiver is both a source of comfort and fear, the child learns to both seek and avoid closeness simultaneously, leading to a confusing mix of emotions and behaviors.

A key feature of disorganized attachment is the lack of a coherent strategy for seeking comfort or security. During times of distress, individuals with this attachment style might show a blend of avoidant and anxious behaviors.

They may seek closeness desperately, only to pull away suddenly when it's offered. They might freeze or dissociate, overwhelmed by their emotions.

These seemingly contradictory behaviors are not signs of manipulation or ill intent, but rather a result of a deep-seated fear of both intimacy and abandonment.

Understanding where disorganized attachment comes from is essential for beginning the healing process. Research indicates that this attachment style often develops from early childhood experiences marked by unpredictability, trauma, or neglect.

When caregivers are emotionally unavailable, abusive, or neglectful, they create an environment where a child's need for safety and connection is met with fear and confusion. This leads to a fragmented view of relationships, resulting in a pervasive sense of insecurity and mistrust.

Disorganized attachment is more common than you might expect and is not a flaw in character or a sign of weakness. It's a natural reaction to challenging circumstances. Although the effects can be profound and long-lasting, healing is achievable.

THE IMPACT OF DISORGANIZED ATTACHMENT

Imagine a child who craves the warmth and comfort of a caregiver's embrace, only to be met with unpredictable responses. One moment, they experience affection and reassurance, and the next, they face withdrawal or even hostility.

This inconsistent interplay of closeness and distance leaves the child feeling confused and insecure, their internal compass spinning in disarray.

As we grow, these early experiences embed themselves deeply into our emotional framework, influencing our expectations of ourselves and others.

We may find ourselves caught in a tug-of-war between a strong desire for connection and a deep fear of intimacy.

Trust becomes a delicate balancing act, constantly at risk of being undermined by fears of rejection or abandonment.

These emotional struggles often play out in our relationships, whether romantic or platonic. We might swing between desperately clinging to loved ones and pushing them away, driven by a deep-seated fear of closeness. Communicating our needs can be a challenge, and we may interpret others' actions through a filter of suspicion and insecurity.

The effects of disorganized attachment go beyond just relationships. They can disrupt our emotional regulation, leading to intense mood swings, anxiety, and even depression. We might find it hard to manage stress, turn to unhealthy coping methods, or feel overwhelmed by the intensity of our emotions.

In some cases, the emotional impact of disorganized attachment can escalate into more severe conditions like post-traumatic stress disorder (PTSD) or complex trauma. These conditions can include symptoms such as flashbacks, nightmares, and a heightened sense of danger, making it challenging to feel safe and secure in the world.

E
X
E
R
C
I
S
E

Create a timeline of your life, marking significant relationships and experiences that may have influenced your attachment style. Reflect on how these events have shaped your current emotional responses and attachment behaviors.

Step-by-Step Instructions

Gather Your Materials:

- Materials Needed: Paper and pen (or a digital tool like a word processor or spreadsheet).

Draw Your Timeline:

- Action: On your paper or digital tool, draw a horizontal line across the page. This line represents your life from birth to the present day.
- Label: Mark key ages or periods along the line (e.g., 0-5 years, 6-10 years, 11-15 years, etc.).

Identify Significant Events:

- Action: For each marked period on your timeline, list significant relationships and experiences. These might include:

- Relationships with family members (e.g., parents, siblings).
- Key events (e.g., moving to a new place, starting school, family changes).
- Important interactions (e.g., friendships, significant caregivers).

Describe Each Event:

- Action: Write a brief description of each significant event or relationship. Include details such as:

What happened during this time.

How the people involved acted toward you.

Any feelings or reactions you had.

Reflect on Impact:

- Action: For each event or relationship, think about how it might have influenced your attachment style. Ask yourself:

Did this event or relationship make me feel secure or insecure?

How did it affect how I relate to others now?

23

Analyze Patterns:

- Action: Look over your timeline and note any patterns. For example:

Are there periods where you felt especially secure or insecure?

Did certain types of experiences (e.g., unpredictability, lack of support) seem to occur more frequently?

Use the template below for this effect or use it as a guide to create yours.

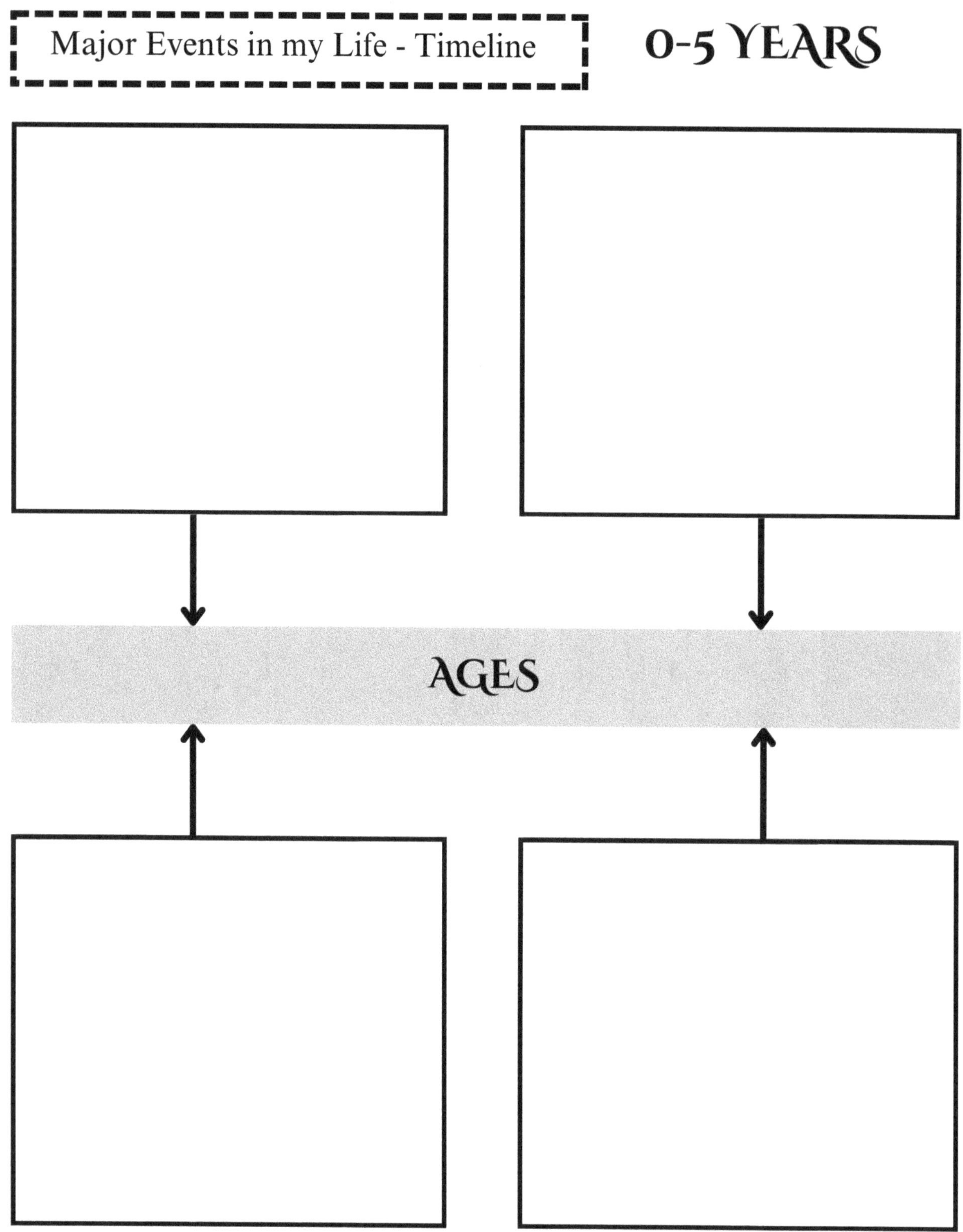

Major Events in my Life - Timeline
0-5 YEARS
AGES

Major Events in my Life - Timeline

6-10 YEARS

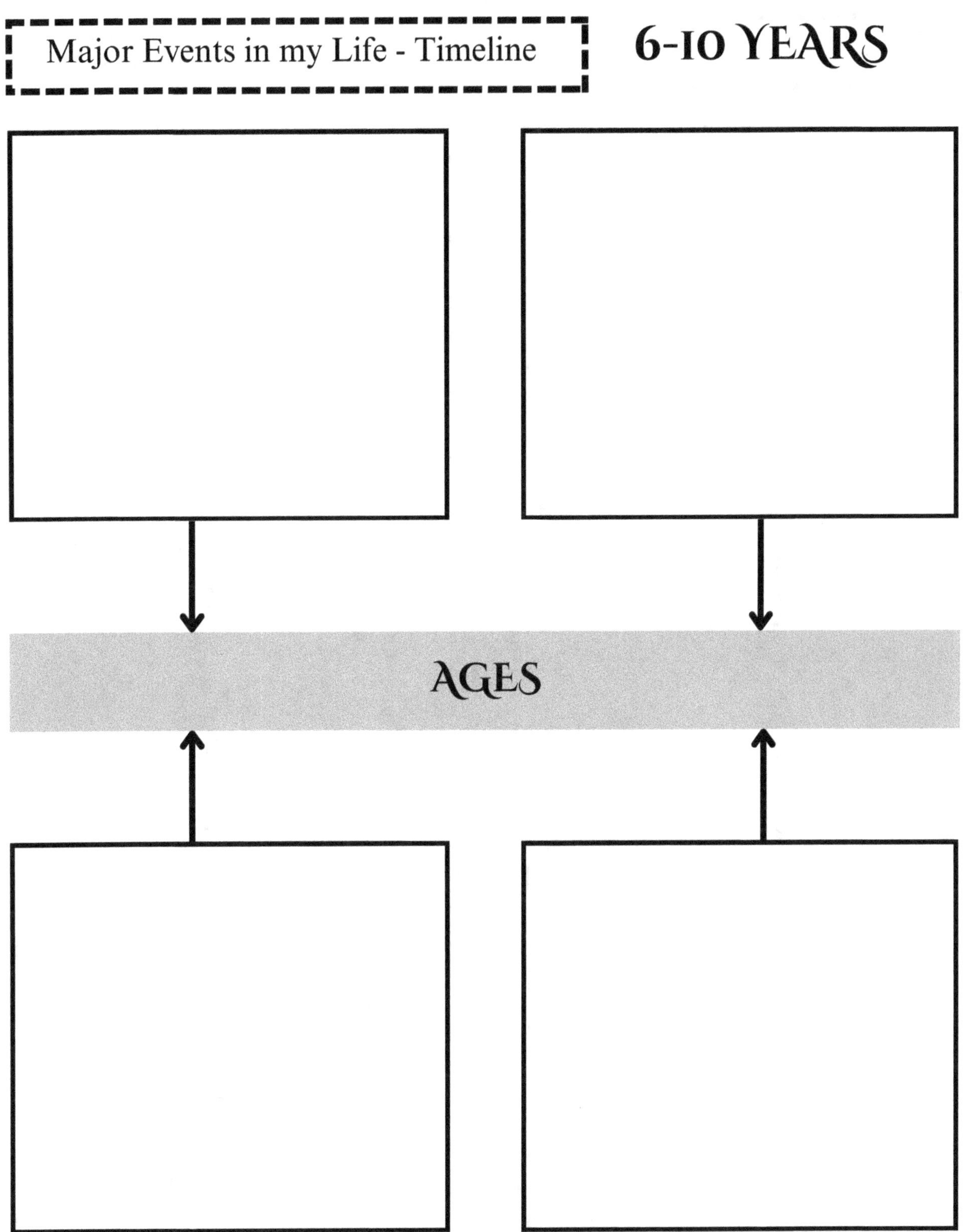

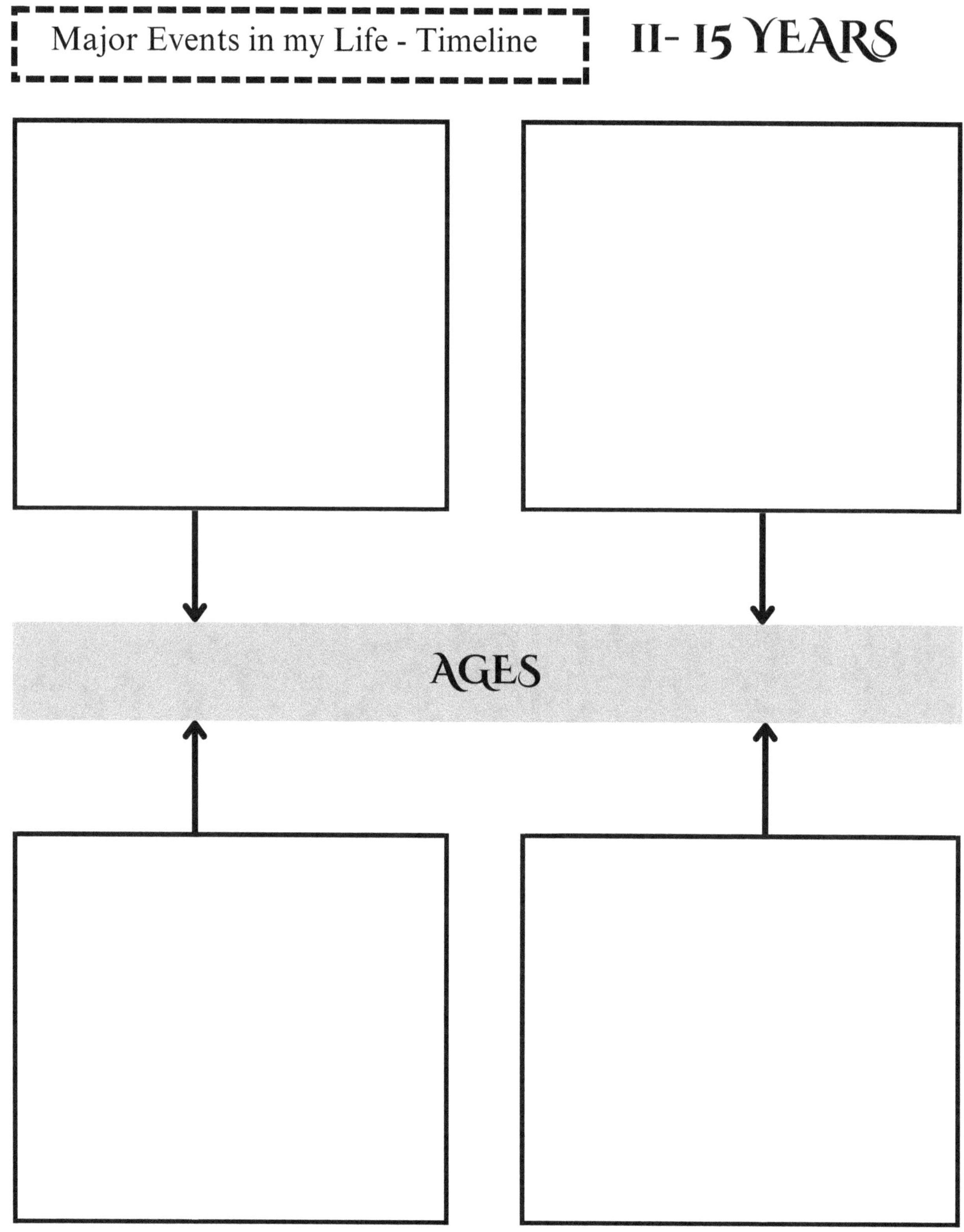
Major Events in my Life - Timeline
11- 15 YEARS
AGES

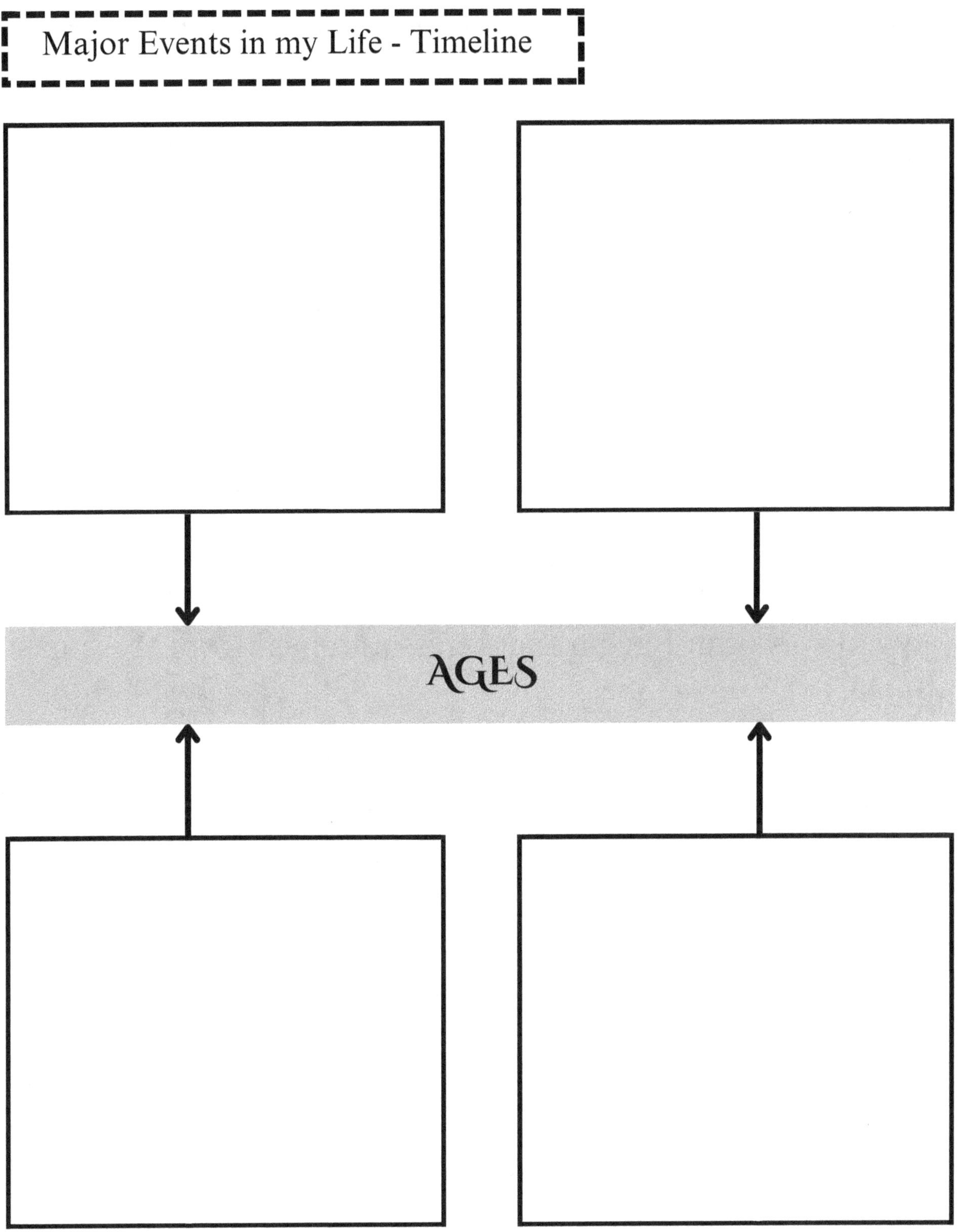
Major Events in my Life - Timeline
AGES

How does my attachment style influence my current relationships and emotional well-being?

____

____

____

____

____

In what ways can I begin to address and heal from these past influences?

____

____

____

____

____

Chapter 2

MENDING EMOTIONAL SCARS

Claire and I had been working together for several months when she experienced a significant breakthrough in our sessions. She had always been open about her struggles with self-esteem and emotional disconnection, but the root of these issues remained elusive.

During our therapy sessions, Claire was consistently frustrated by her inability to understand why she felt so inadequate despite her many accomplishments.

Everything changed one chilly afternoon in November. Claire's family had gathered for a memorial service to honor her recently deceased mother. The atmosphere was somber, and the small, cozy church in Seattle was filled with relatives and old family friends sharing their memories.

As Claire was going through her mother's belongings in the old family home later that day, she stumbled upon a collection of dusty, handwritten letters hidden in a forgotten drawer.

Curiosity piqued, Claire began to read the letters, and her world shifted. The letters were from her mother's younger years, written to a close friend who had since passed away. They detailed a harrowing account of her mother's own childhood—years of neglect and emotional abuse from her parents, who had been unable to offer the love and support a child needs.

Claire's mother had written candidly about her feelings of abandonment and her desperate attempts to shield Claire from the same pain.

The twist came when Claire discovered that the letters contained not only her mother's raw emotions but also her mother's regrets and sorrow about repeating some of those harmful patterns with Claire.

Her mother had tried to protect her from the same type of emotional neglect she had endured, but in doing so, had inadvertently created a different kind of emotional distance. Claire felt a mix of anger and sadness as she realized that her mother's attempts to shield her had actually deepened the emotional rift between them.

The revelation hit Claire like a tidal wave. It was both devastating and enlightening.

The realization that her mother's behavior was a reflection of her own unresolved trauma rather than a personal failing on Claire's part gave her a new perspective on her family dynamics. Claire's emotional pain was not just a result of her own inadequacies but a complex legacy of intergenerational trauma.

This discovery became a turning point for Claire. She began to see her mother's actions through the lens of empathy and understanding rather than solely as personal betrayals.

As Claire processed these newly uncovered emotions, she found herself gradually letting go of her own self-blame and embracing self-compassion.

Emotional scars, like physical ones, are evidence of a life lived with depth, love, and experience. However, unlike the physical wounds that eventually fade, the emotional injuries we carry can persist, influencing our thoughts, behaviors, and relationships.

If your childhood was marked by inconsistent caregiving, neglect, or trauma, you may be dealing with the effects of disorganized attachment. This attachment style, shaped by a chaotic upbringing, often leaves individuals feeling lost, disconnected, and uncertain of their place in the world.

But it's important to remember that these emotional scars, while painful, do not define you. They are not a permanent sentence but an opportunity for healing and growth.

Think of your emotional scars as lines on a weathered map, each one symbolizing a path you've traveled and a challenge you've overcome.

They are a testament to your strength, resilience, and ability to endure. The journey to healing these scars may be difficult, but it is unquestionably worth the effort.

Start by acknowledging the depth of your wounds. Allow yourself to feel the pain, anger, and confusion that lie within. Suppressing these emotions only buries them deeper, hindering the healing process. Embrace the discomfort as an essential step toward freedom.

Just as a skilled surgeon carefully stitches a wound, you too must learn to mend the pieces of your heart. This involves confronting the memories and experiences that have shaped your attachment style.

Through therapy, journaling, or other forms of self-expression, you can gently untangle the threads of your past and weave them into a story of strength and resilience.

Remember that healing is not a straightforward journey. There will be setbacks, moments of doubt, and times when old wounds resurface.

Be patient with yourself, and don't hesitate to seek support from therapists, support groups, or trusted loved ones. Their guidance and empathy can be invaluable as you navigate this challenging path.

Forgiveness, both of yourself and those who have hurt you, is a vital part of the healing process. This doesn't mean excusing harmful actions, but rather letting go of the resentment that weighs you down. Forgiveness is an act of self-love, allowing you to move forward with a lighter heart.

As you work through your emotional scars, you'll develop a deeper sense of self-awareness and compassion. You'll learn to recognize your triggers, establish healthy boundaries, and communicate your needs effectively. These skills are essential for building and maintaining healthy relationships, both with yourself and others.

Healing from emotional scars isn't about erasing the past but transforming it. It's about finding meaning in your experiences, learning from your mistakes, and using your pain as a catalyst for growth. Remember, you are not alone on this journey. Many others have walked this path before you, and many more will follow. By sharing your story, you not only heal yourself but also offer hope and inspiration to others.

RECOGNIZING AND PROCESSING DIFFICULT EMOTIONS

Living with disorganized attachment can feel like navigating a turbulent emotional landscape, where highs and lows come without warning. One moment, you might crave closeness with someone, only to recoil the next out of fear of vulnerability or rejection.

You might find yourself suddenly overwhelmed by anger or plunged into deep sadness, leaving you feeling isolated and alone.

These intense emotional swings can be exhausting and disorienting, but it's important to understand that they are not signs of weakness or failure.

Instead, they reflect your natural response to the difficult experiences you've endured.

Understanding the origins of these emotions is a key step in your healing journey. Disorganized attachment often develops in response to inconsistent or frightening caregiving during childhood.

When the people you relied on for safety and comfort were unpredictable or emotionally unavailable, you might have learned to suppress your emotions or express them in ways that felt chaotic and out of control. As a result, you may now feel disconnected from your emotions, making it difficult to recognize and manage them effectively.

The good news is that you can learn to navigate your emotions in a healthier way. The first step is to become more aware of your emotional state. Set aside time each day to check in with yourself and notice what you're feeling. Instead of judging or suppressing your emotions, acknowledge them as they arise.

You might say to yourself, "I'm feeling anxious right now," or "I'm feeling a wave of sadness." This simple act of naming your emotions can help you regain a sense of control over them.

It's also beneficial to pay attention to the physical sensations that accompany your emotions. For example, when you're feeling anxious, you might notice your heart beating faster, your palms getting sweaty, or a tight feeling in your stomach.

When you're sad, you might feel a heaviness in your chest or a lump in your throat. By tuning into these physical cues, you can gain a better understanding of what you're feeling emotionally.

As you become more skilled at identifying your emotions, you can start to explore their underlying causes. What triggers certain feelings? Are there patterns or recurring themes in your emotional responses?

DEVELOPING SELF-COMPASSION AND ACCEPTANCE

Disorganized attachment can indeed cast long, lingering shadows, leaving you feeling fragmented and uncertain about your place in the world. You may have spent years grappling with a whirlwind of emotions—fear, anger, sadness, and a deep, gnawing sense of emptiness.

These feelings are not your fault; they are the legacy of experiences that taught you the world wasn't always a safe or predictable place. But here's an essential truth: those experiences, as powerful as they may be, do not define you.

Beneath the layers of hurt, confusion, and pain lies your true self—a self that is whole, resilient, and capable of profound love and connection. Uncovering this self requires a journey of self-compassion.

This journey is not about ignoring the pain or indulging in self-pity. Instead, it's about embracing every part of who you are, even the parts that hurt the most.

Think of self-compassion as a warm embrace on a cold day. It involves recognizing your struggles without judgment and offering yourself the same kindness and understanding you would offer a close friend.

When you stumble or make mistakes, self-compassion gently reminds you, "It's okay. You're human. You're learning and growing." Your worth isn't tied to perfection but to your willingness to show up for yourself with an open heart.

A practical way to cultivate self-compassion is by challenging the critical voice that often echoes in your mind. This voice may tell you that you're not good enough, that you're unlovable, or that you'll never heal. But remember, this voice isn't the truth; it's a distortion shaped by past wounds.

When you hear this voice, gently acknowledge it, then counter it with affirmations of self-worth and kindness.

Acceptance is another key part of this healing process. Accepting your past doesn't mean condoning the hurt you've experienced;

instead, it means acknowledging that it happened and allowing yourself to feel the full range of emotions that come with it. It's about releasing the need to change or deny your history and choosing instead to learn and grow from it.

As you practice self-compassion and acceptance, you may notice a gradual shift within yourself. The sharp edges of your pain might begin to soften, replaced by a sense of peace and understanding. You'll start to see yourself not as a collection of broken pieces, but as a whole, complex being with the capacity to heal and thrive.

Remember, this journey is a process, not a destination. There will be days when self-compassion comes easily and days when it feels like a struggle. Be patient with yourself and keep showing up. Every act of kindness towards yourself, no matter how small, is a step towards wholeness.

Your past may have conditioned you to see yourself through a lens of fear and insecurity, but with self-compassion and acceptance, you can rewrite that narrative.

E X E R C I S E

Keep a daily journal where you write about your emotions, particularly focusing on difficult or overwhelming feelings. Reflect on the triggers and the thoughts that accompany these emotions. Over time, notice any patterns that emerge.

Step-by-Step Instructions

Set Up Your Journal:

- Materials Needed: A notebook, journal, or a digital tool like a notes app or word processor.
- Action: Designate a specific place where you will write about your emotions daily. It could be a physical journal or an app on your phone —whatever feels most comfortable for you.

Choose a Time to Write:

- Action: Decide on a regular time each day to write in your journal. This could be in the morning, before bed, or at any time that fits into your routine. Consistency is key to making this exercise effective.

Reflect on Your Day:

- Action: At your chosen time, take a few moments to think about your day. Ask yourself:

What emotions did I experience today?

Were there any moments when I felt particularly strong emotions, like sadness, anger, anxiety, or joy?

Write About Your Emotions:

- Action: Write down the emotions you felt during the day. Be as specific as possible (e.g., "I felt frustrated when my friend canceled our plans" instead of just "I felt bad").
- Include Details: Describe the situation that triggered the emotion. What was happening? Who was involved? What thoughts crossed your mind at that moment?

Explore the Triggers:

- Action: Reflect on what might have triggered the emotion. Consider:

Was it something someone said or did?

Was it a situation that reminded you of a past experience?

Did a specific thought or worry come up that made the emotion stronger?

Notice Accompanying Thoughts:

- Action: Write down any thoughts that came up alongside the emotion. For example:

If you felt anxious, what were you worried about?

If you felt angry, what thoughts were running through your mind?

Question: Ask yourself if these thoughts were based on facts, assumptions, or fears.

Look for Patterns Over Time:

- Action: After a week or two, review your journal entries. Look for any patterns:

Are there certain emotions you experience more often?

Do certain triggers or situations keep coming up?

Are there recurring thoughts that seem to amplify your emotions?

Reflect and Adjust:

- Action: As you begin to notice patterns, think about how they affect your life. Are there changes you can make to manage your emotions more effectively? For example:

If you notice that you often feel stressed about work, could you find ways to reduce that stress?

If certain thoughts are making your emotions worse, could you challenge or reframe those thoughts?

Celebrate Your Progress:
- Action: Acknowledge any insights or improvements you've made. Keeping an emotion journal is a valuable tool for self-awareness and emotional healing. Celebrate small wins, like recognizing a pattern or managing a difficult emotion better than before.

Keep Going:
- Action: Continue journaling regularly. The more you practice, the better you'll become at understanding and managing your emotions.

Register Your Emotions here

Date

Trigger for
this emotion

Ways I can
work on this
emotions

Register Your Emotions here

Date

Trigger for
this emotion

Ways I can
work on this
emotions

Register Your Emotions here

Date

Trigger for
this emotion

Ways I can
work on this
emotions

Register Your Emotions here

Date

Trigger for
this emotion

Ways I can
work on this
emotions

Register Your Emotions here

Date

Trigger for
this emotion

Ways I can
work on this
emotions

How can I practice self-compassion when facing difficult emotions?

____

____

____

____

What steps can I take to accept my emotions rather than avoid or suppress them?

____

____

____

____

Chapter 3

FOSTERING RESILIENCE

Daniel came to me in his late twenties, his face etched with the kind of tension that never really goes away. He had grown up in a small town in Oregon, a place where everyone knew each other and where secrets were nearly impossible to keep.

His father, a mechanic who owned the only garage in town, was well-known for his skill with engines and his unpredictable temper. When things were good, they were really good.

Daniel's father would spend hours teaching him how to fix cars, patiently explaining the intricacies of each part, sharing stories from his own childhood, and laughing over dinner. But when things were bad, the house felt like a powder keg waiting to explode.

Daniel described how his father's mood could change with the weather, or so it seemed. A tough day at the garage, a problem with a customer, or just a wrong look from someone could set him off.

When he was in one of his darker moods, he would withdraw completely, retreating to the garage and leaving Daniel and his mother to tiptoe around the house, afraid to disturb him.

At times, his frustration would boil over, and he would lash out verbally, saying things that stung deeply and left Daniel questioning his own worth. The worst part was the unpredictability of it all—Daniel never knew which version of his father he would come home to.

As a child, Daniel learned to brace himself whenever he heard the sound of his father's truck pulling into the driveway. If the engine revved a little too loudly, he knew to keep his distance.

If it purred softly, he might dare to approach, hoping to catch a glimpse of the father who would ruffle his hair and call him "buddy."

This constant state of vigilance took its toll. By the time he was a teenager, Daniel had developed a knack for reading people's moods, a skill he honed out of necessity. But this ability to sense the emotional undercurrents in a room didn't bring him peace; instead, it fed his anxiety, making him feel like he was always walking on eggshells.

When Daniel came to see me, he was struggling with intense anxiety and frequent panic attacks. He described feeling like he was constantly on edge, never able to fully relax, even in situations that were supposed to be enjoyable.

He had a good job as a graphic designer, but he often found himself paralyzed by self-doubt, fearing that any mistake could lead to catastrophic consequences.

In relationships, he was quick to apologize, even when he hadn't done anything wrong, just to avoid the possibility of conflict.

He was exhausted, both physically and emotionally, from the constant effort it took to keep everything in his life under control.

We began our work together by exploring the roots of his anxiety, tracing it back to those early experiences with his father.

It became clear that Daniel's nervous system had been conditioned to operate in a state of hyper-vigilance, always ready to react to the slightest hint of danger. He had never learned how to regulate his emotions because he had never been in an environment where it felt safe to let his guard down.

His father's unpredictable behavior had left him feeling like he had to be prepared for anything at any moment, a habit that had carried over into every aspect of his adult life.

Resilience isn't about being unbreakable or avoiding pain. It's about recognizing the pain, embracing the challenges, and having the courage to keep going.

Think of resilience as a muscle that grows stronger with use and weakens if neglected. For those of us who grew up with disorganized attachment, this muscle might not have been well-developed in our early years.

The inconsistent, unpredictable, or even frightening caregiving we experienced may have left us feeling vulnerable and unprepared to face life's inevitable hardships.

It's never too late to start building resilience. Research shows that our brains are incredibly adaptable, capable of rewiring and forming new neural connections throughout our lives. This means that even if our early experiences didn't nurture resilience, we can still develop it through intentional effort and practice.

So, what does it mean to build resilience? It's a complex process that involves developing a range of skills and practices.

It means learning to regulate our emotions, identify and manage triggers, develop healthy coping strategies, and build a strong support network.

It also involves cultivating self-compassion, recognizing our strengths, and accepting our imperfections.

Imagine resilience as a toolbox filled with various tools. Some of these tools are practical, like learning relaxation techniques or establishing healthy routines.

Others are emotional, like practicing self-compassion or challenging negative self-talk. And some are relational, like seeking support from loved ones or building a community of supportive individuals.

The specific tools that work for each of us might differ, and that's okay. The key is to experiment and find the ones that resonate with you. It's also important to remember that building resilience is an ongoing process.

There will be setbacks and challenges, but with persistence and a willingness to learn, you can grow stronger and more resilient over time.

BUILDING EMOTIONAL REGULATION SKILLS

Emotional regulation isn't about pushing your feelings aside; it's about recognizing, understanding, and responding to them in a healthy way.

This skill is essential for anyone aiming to live a more balanced and fulfilling life, especially for those who've faced the specific challenges that come with disorganized attachment.

Imagine your emotions as messengers, each delivering important information about your needs, boundaries, and overall well-being.

For those with disorganized attachment, these messages might come through in a confusing or overwhelming way.

You might experience intense emotional swings, react impulsively, or struggle to accurately identify and express your feelings. This is why developing emotional regulation skills is so important.

Let's move into a key skill that can support you on this journey:

Mindfulness: At its essence, mindfulness is about being present in the moment without judgment. It involves noticing your thoughts and feelings as they come up, without getting swept away by them. By practicing mindfulness, you create a gap between yourself and your emotions, which allows you to respond thoughtfully rather than reacting on impulse.

Practice: Dedicate a few minutes each day to sitting quietly and focusing on your breath. Pay attention to the sensations in your body and the thoughts that drift through your mind. When you notice your attention wandering, gently guide it back to your breath. Over time, this practice will help you become more in tune with your emotional landscape.

E X E R C I S E

Choose a Quiet Space:

- Action: Find a calm and quiet place where you won't be disturbed. This could be a cozy corner of your home, a quiet park, or any spot where you feel relaxed.

Get Comfortable:

- Action: Sit or lie down in a comfortable position. Ensure your body is relaxed and your posture is upright but not tense. You can use a chair, cushion, or the floor—whatever feels best for you.

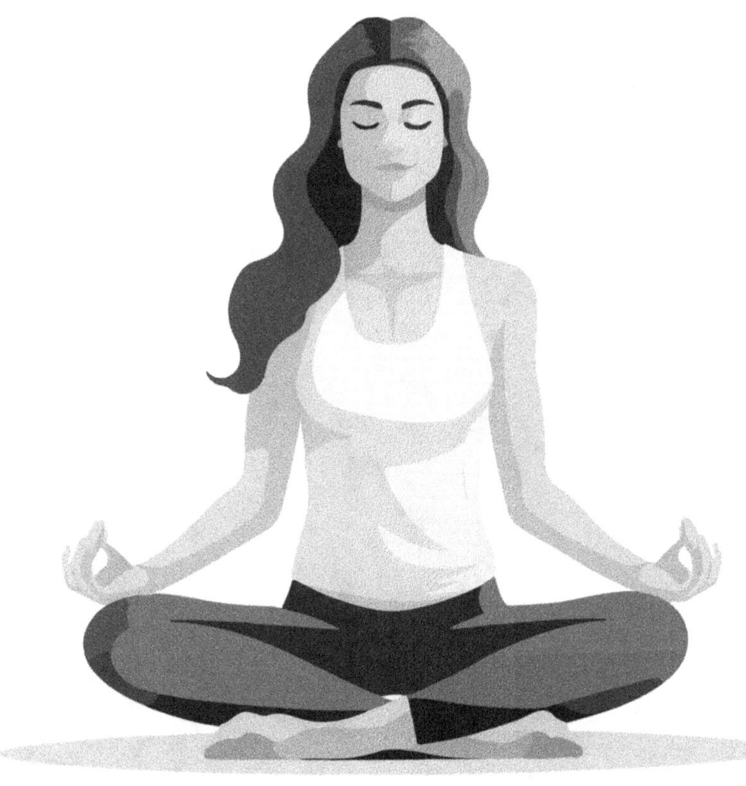

Close Your Eyes:

- Action: Gently close your eyes to minimize distractions. This helps you focus better on your breath and the sensations in your body.

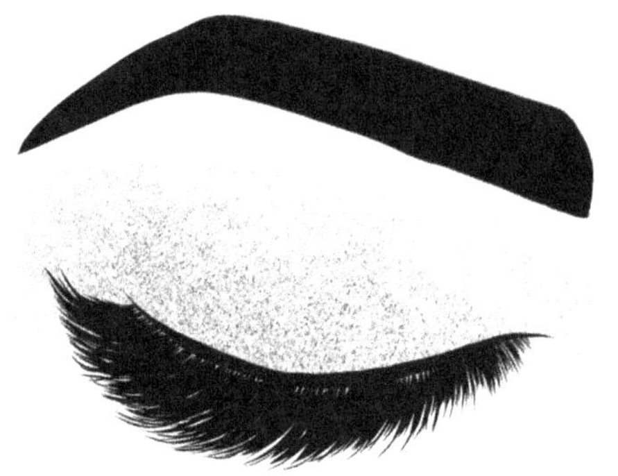 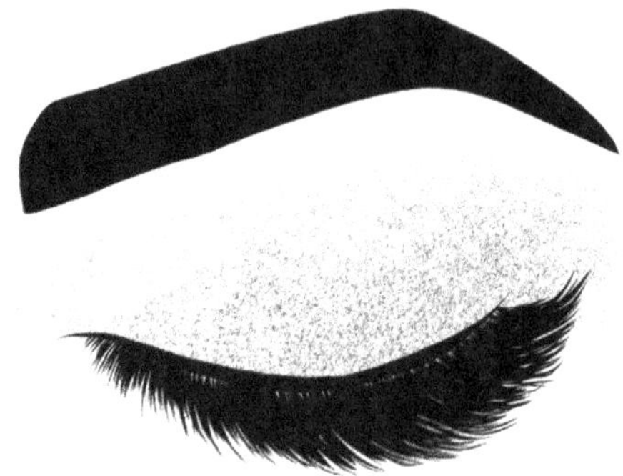

Take a Deep Breath:

- Action: Begin by taking a deep breath in through your nose. Allow your belly to expand as you inhale deeply, filling your lungs with air. Hold the breath for a moment.

Exhale Slowly:

- Action: Breathe out slowly and completely through your mouth or nose. Pay attention to the sensation of the air leaving your body. Notice any tension releasing as you exhale.

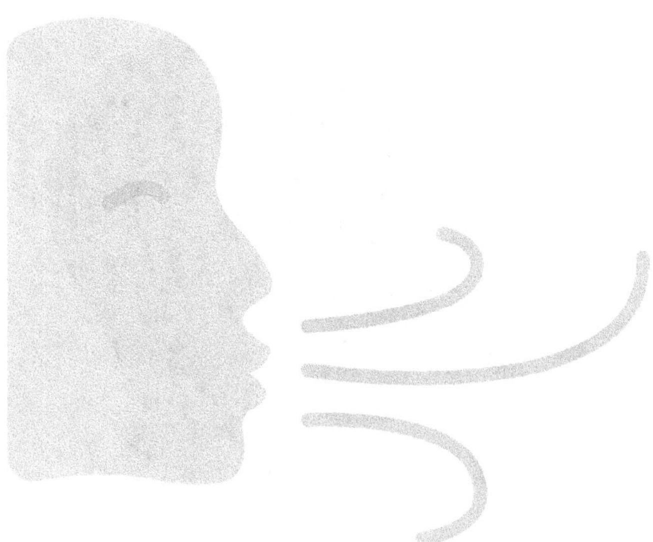

Focus on Your Breathing:

- Action: Continue to breathe naturally, focusing your attention on the rhythm of your breath. Notice the feeling of the air entering and leaving your nostrils, the rise and fall of your chest, or the gentle expansion and contraction of your belly.

Observe Without Judgment:

- Action: As you breathe, thoughts or distractions might arise. When they do, gently bring your focus back to your breath. It's normal for your mind to wander—just acknowledge it and return to observing your breath.

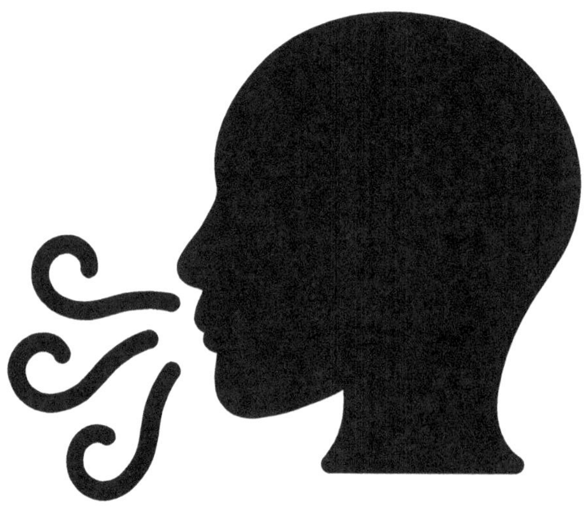

Set a Timer:

- Action: Use a timer to keep track of the time. Start with 5 minutes and gradually increase to 10 minutes as you become more comfortable with the practice.

Reflect on the Experience:

- Action: After your mindful breathing session, take a moment to reflect on how you feel. Notice any changes in your mood or physical sensations. Appreciate the calm and focus you've created through this practice.

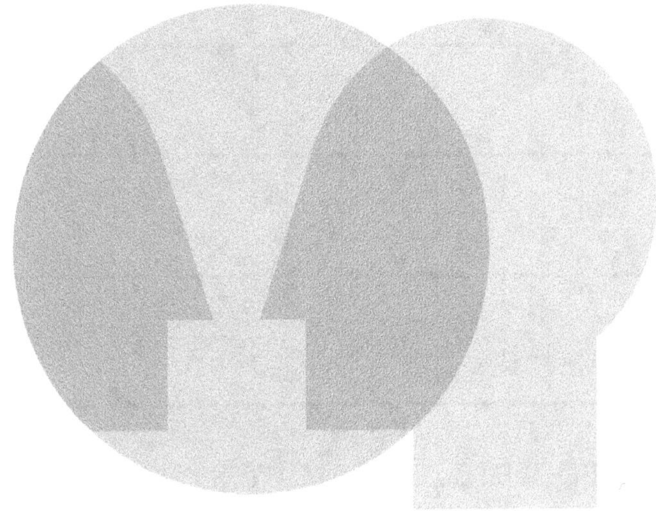

Make It a Daily Habit:

- Action: Incorporate mindful breathing into your daily routine. Choose a specific time each day, such as in the morning, during a break, or before bed, to practice consistently.

What challenges do I face when trying to stay present in the moment?

____

____

____

____

How can I incorporate mindfulness into my daily life to build resilience?

____

____

____

____

Chapter 4

NURTURING SECURE RELATIONSHIPS

In my early years as a therapist, I worked with a client named Alan. He was in his mid-thirties, a successful architect based in San Francisco, known for his meticulous designs and innovative ideas.

On the surface, Alan had everything going for him—he was well-respected in his field, had a close-knit group of friends, and seemed to lead a fulfilling life.

But beneath this exterior, Alan was deeply troubled by his inability to maintain romantic relationships.

Every time he started to feel close to someone, he would find himself pulling away, distancing himself emotionally until the relationship inevitably fell apart.

Alan's pattern of intense closeness followed by sudden withdrawal puzzled him.

He desperately wanted to connect with someone on a deeper level, to experience the kind of love and partnership he saw in others around him.

Yet, no matter how hard he tried, something always held him back. It was as though an invisible barrier prevented him from fully trusting anyone, from allowing himself to be vulnerable.

As we dug into Alan's past during our sessions, a clearer picture began to emerge. Alan grew up in a household that was, on the surface, stable and supportive. His father was a well-known attorney, stern but fair, while his mother was the epitome of grace, always ensuring their home was warm and inviting.

But this idyllic image masked a much darker reality. Alan's father had a temper—an explosive, unpredictable anger that could be triggered by the smallest of things. A misplaced toy, a minor inconvenience, anything could set him off.

These outbursts were rare, but when they happened, they were terrifying.

As a child, Alan never knew which version of his father he would encounter. The loving dad who taught him how to ride a bike or the terrifying figure who would scream and break things in a blind rage.

The inconsistency created a constant state of anxiety in Alan, a fear that kept him on edge, always trying to anticipate and avoid his father's wrath.

His mother, though kind, was often passive in the face of these outbursts, urging Alan to "stay out of your father's way" rather than confronting the problem.

This childhood environment left Alan deeply scarred. The love he received from his father was conditional, and it came with an undercurrent of fear. As he grew older, Alan unconsciously carried this fear into his adult relationships.

The closer he became to someone, the more he feared the potential for pain, rejection, or betrayal.

To protect himself, he would withdraw emotionally, cutting off his feelings before anyone could hurt him.

One particular relationship stood out in our conversations —a woman named Catherine. Alan had met Catherine at a gallery opening in the city. She was an artist, free-spirited and full of life, the complete opposite of Alan's meticulous, controlled nature.

They were drawn to each other almost immediately, and their relationship developed quickly. For a while, everything seemed perfect. Alan felt more connected to Catherine than he had to anyone in years. But as their relationship deepened, so did his anxiety.

He began to notice small things that would trigger his fear —a certain tone in Catherine's voice, a look she gave him when she was upset. These were echoes of his father's unpredictable anger, and they terrified him.

Alan began to pull away, inventing reasons to avoid spending time with Catherine. He buried himself in work, stayed late at the office, and became distant and aloof.

Catherine, hurt and confused, tried to reach out to him, but the more she tried, the more Alan retreated. Eventually, the relationship ended, not with a fight, but with a slow, painful drift into silence. Alan was left alone, once again wondering why he couldn't make love work.

Through our sessions, Alan began to understand that his fear wasn't about Catherine or any of the women he had dated. It was about the unresolved trauma from his childhood, the fear of love turning into pain that he had experienced with his father.

This realization was both painful and liberating for Alan. It wasn't an immediate fix, but it was the first step towards healing.

Building secure relationships involves facing your fears, questioning your assumptions, and developing new ways of connecting with others. It's a journey of self-discovery, compassion, and ultimately, empowerment.

With the help of therapy, self-reflection, and intentional effort, you can learn to regulate your emotions, establish trust, and cultivate healthy, fulfilling connections.

Picture a life where relationships feel safe, supportive, and enriching. A life where you can express your emotions freely, without the fear of judgment or rejection.

A life where you can rely on others for support and offer your own love and compassion in return. This is the promise of secure attachment, and it's within your grasp.

The path to healing isn't always easy. It may involve confronting painful memories, questioning deeply held beliefs, and stepping outside your comfort zone.

But with patience, perseverance, and the right support, you can create lasting change and build relationships that truly nourish your soul.

UNDERSTANDING HEALTHY RELATIONSHIP DYNAMICS

Have you ever looked at a seemingly happy couple and wondered, "How do they make it work?" The reality is that healthy relationships aren't a matter of luck or fairy tale magic.

They're built on understanding, effort, and shared growth. Grasping the dynamics of a healthy relationship is like having a guide to navigate the often complex landscape of connecting with another person.

Disorganized attachment style can make it difficult to trust others, regulate emotions, and form secure connections. However, this doesn't mean that healthy relationships are out of reach.

Think of it this way: imagine you've spent years walking a winding path through a dense forest. It's familiar, but it's not always easy, and you often find yourself lost or unsure of the way forward. Understanding healthy relationship dynamics is like stepping out of that forest and into a clearing.

The path ahead might still have its twists and turns, but you now have a clearer view, more sunlight, and the tools to navigate with confidence.

So, what does a healthy relationship look like? It's not about perfection or never having disagreements.

It's about feeling safe enough to be yourself, to express your needs and feelings without the fear of judgment or rejection. It's about having someone who truly listens to you, respects your boundaries, and supports your growth.

One of the most critical elements of a healthy relationship is trust. Trust doesn't develop overnight; it requires consistent effort from both partners.

Trust means believing that the other person has your best interests at heart, even during disagreements.

It means feeling secure enough to be vulnerable, knowing that your feelings and needs will be respected.

Communication is another vital foundation of a healthy relationship. This goes beyond just talking; it's about truly listening and understanding each other. It's about being able to express your thoughts and feelings honestly, even when it's tough, and knowing that your partner will listen with an open mind and heart.

Healthy relationships also allow for individuality and growth. It's not about losing yourself in your partner, but rather about supporting each other's dreams and aspirations. It's about celebrating each other's successes and offering comfort and encouragement during challenges.

For those with disorganized attachment, understanding healthy relationship dynamics can be life-changing. It offers a new perspective on your own behaviors and reactions, as well as those of your partner. It provides the tools to communicate more effectively, build trust, and create a relationship that feels safe and supportive.

BUILDING TRUST AND COMMUNICATION SKILLS

The foundation of any healthy relationship, whether romantic, familial, or a friendship, is built on trust and communication.

If you have a disorganized attachment style, these pillars might feel particularly challenging to establish. But just as a house can be rebuilt after a storm, your relationships can be reconstructed with care and effort.

So, how do you begin to rebuild trust? Start by taking small, manageable risks. Share something personal with a trusted friend or family member.

Open up about your feelings and vulnerabilities. If they respond with empathy and support, it will reinforce your belief in their trustworthiness. Trust, much like a muscle, grows stronger with consistent use.

Communication is equally crucial. It's the bridge that connects us to others, allowing us to express our thoughts, feelings, and needs.

However, if you have disorganized attachment, communication can sometimes feel like navigating a minefield. You may worry about saying the wrong thing, being misunderstood, or even facing rejection. Yet, healthy communication is essential for resolving conflicts, deepening intimacy, and building stronger connections.

A good starting point is practicing active listening. When someone is speaking, give them your full attention. Nod your head, maintain eye contact, and reflect back what you hear.

This shows that you're not just hearing their words, but also understanding their emotions. Remember, communication is a two-way street. It's not just about expressing yourself; it's also about truly listening to and understanding others.

By focusing on these foundational aspects—trust and communication—you can begin to rebuild your relationships, creating a stronger, more secure connection with those around you.

EXERCISE

Schedule regular check-ins with a trusted person in your life. During these check-ins, practice open communication, expressing your needs, and listening without judgment. Reflect on the dynamics of these interactions.

Step 1: Choose a Trusted Person

- Action: Identify someone you feel comfortable with and trust, such as a close friend, family member, or partner. This should be someone who supports your growth and is open to engaging in meaningful conversations.

Step 2: Schedule Regular Check-Ins

- Action: Agree on a specific time and frequency for your check-ins. It could be once a week, bi-weekly, or monthly—whatever works best for both of you. Set a reminder or add it to your calendar to ensure consistency.
- Example: "Every Sunday evening at 7 PM" or "The first Saturday of every month."

Step 3: Prepare for the Conversation

- Action: Before each check-in, take a few minutes to think about what you want to discuss. Consider any needs, concerns, or feelings you want to express. It's also helpful to reflect on recent experiences or situations where communication was important.
- Tips:
  - Keep a list of topics if it helps you stay focused.
  - Think about how you can express your thoughts clearly and calmly.

Step 4: Practice Open Communication

- Action: During the check-in, share your thoughts, feelings, and needs openly. Be honest about what's on your mind, but also be mindful of how you communicate—aim for clarity and kindness.
- Example Statements:

"I've been feeling a bit distant lately and wanted to talk about it."

I really appreciate how supportive you've been, and I wanted to acknowledge that."

Step 5: Listen Without Judgment

- Action: When the other person shares their thoughts, practice active listening. This means focusing fully on what they're saying, without interrupting, judging, or planning your response while they're talking.
- Tips:

Nod or provide verbal acknowledgments (e.g., "I understand," "That makes sense").

Ask clarifying questions if needed (e.g., "Can you tell me more about that?").

Step 6: Reflect on the Interaction

- Action: After the conversation, take some time to reflect on how it went. Consider the following:

Did you feel heard and understood?

Were you able to express yourself clearly?

How did the other person respond?

What went well, and what could be improved for next time?

- Journal: Write down your reflections in a journal to track your progress over time. This can help you identify patterns, improvements, and areas where you might want to focus more attention.

Step 7: Adjust and Continue

- Action: Based on your reflections, discuss with your check-in partner if there's anything that can be adjusted for future conversations. Keep the check-ins going as a regular practice to nurture and strengthen your relationship.
- Example Adjustments:

"Let's try to be more specific about our needs next time."

"I think we should set a little more time aside for these talks."

Below is a difficult conversation template to help you on this exercise.

1 *What do you want/need to have this conversation? what do you think will happen?*

2 *How will I start the conversation?*

3 *How will I share my story/feelings?*

4 *What questions can I ask to get their perspective?*

5 *What are some simple solution I can suggest?*

Name

1 *What do you want/need to have this conversation? what do you think will happen?*

2 *How will I start the conversation?*

3 *How will I share my story/feelings?*

4 *What questions can I ask to get their perspective?*

5 *What are some simple solution I can suggest?*

Name

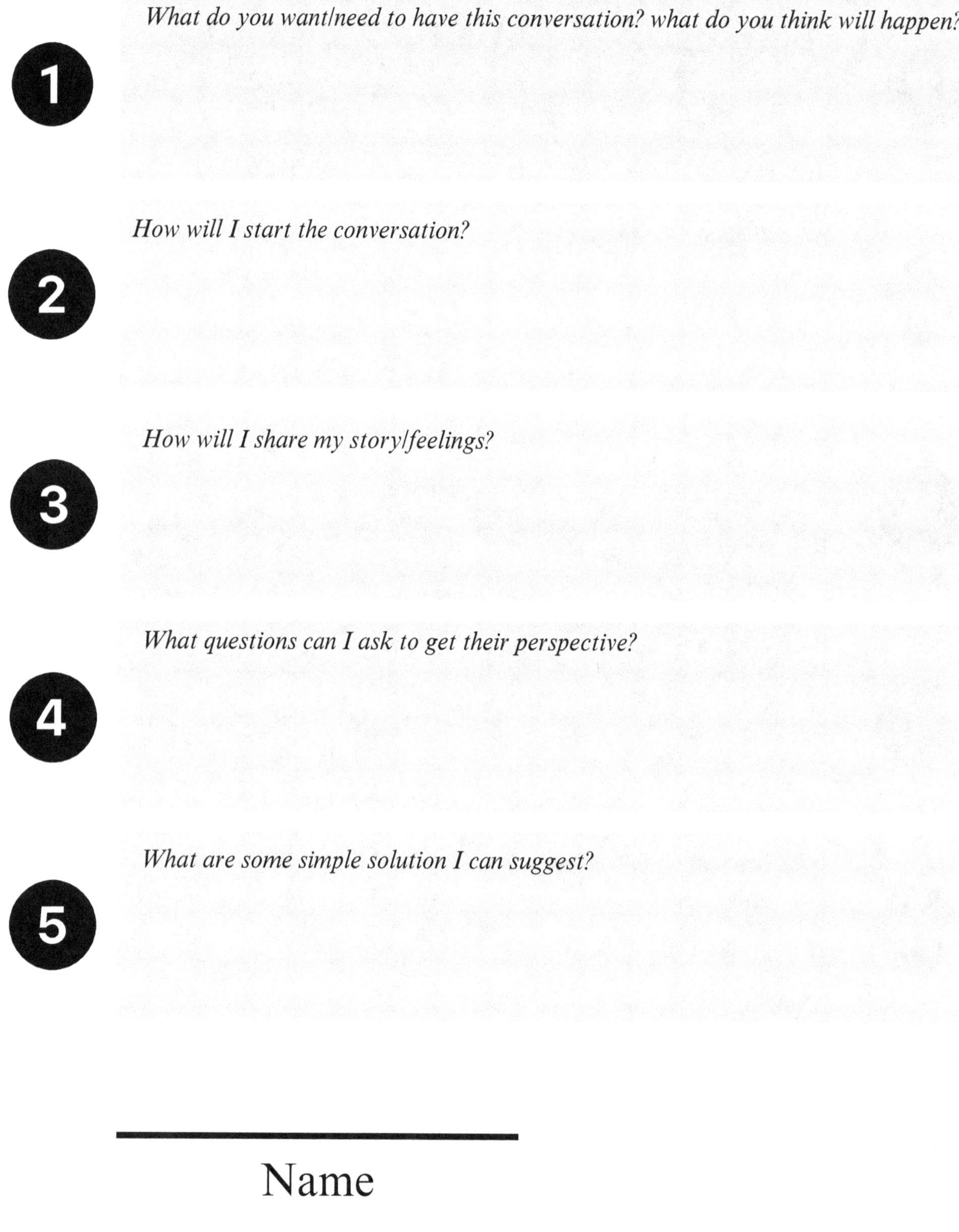

What do you want/need to have this conversation? what do you think will happen?

1

How will I start the conversation?

2

How will I share my story/feelings?

3

What questions can I ask to get their perspective?

4

What are some simple solution I can suggest?

5

Name

What steps can I take to build trust in my relationships?

____

____

____

____

How can I improve my communication skills to foster healthier connections?

____

____

____

____

"The way we relate to others is the way we relate to ourselves." — Peter A. Levine

Chapter 5

HEALING THROUGH SELF-CARE

I vividly remember Carla, a client I worked with in my office in Seattle. She had a background that was nothing short of tumultuous.

Growing up with a mother who struggled with severe depression and substance abuse, Carla had to navigate a chaotic environment that left her feeling neglected and emotionally abandoned.

By the time Carla came to me, she was an adult grappling with feelings of worthlessness and an inability to maintain stable relationships.

Our initial sessions were challenging. Carla's sense of self was fragile, and she had a tendency to self-sabotage whenever things started to improve.

We began by addressing her physical well-being, an area she had long neglected.

I encouraged Carla to start with small, manageable changes: a consistent sleep schedule, regular meals, and integrating some form of exercise into her daily routine.

She decided to start walking every morning at Greenwood Park, a place that had always brought her a bit of solace.

As Carla gradually improved her physical health, we shifted our focus to her emotional and mental well-being. Her past traumas were deeply ingrained, affecting her view of herself and her relationships.

We worked on building self-compassion, which was a new concept for her. She created a self-compassion mantra that she recited daily, something like, "I am worthy of love and care."

At first, she struggled with believing these affirmations, but over time, they began to resonate with her.

One of the more profound moments in our work together came during a particularly tough session. Carla had a breakthrough when she realized how much she had internalized her mother's struggles as a reflection of her own worth.

This was a pivotal moment in our journey. We started to explore healthier ways for her to set boundaries and establish supportive relationships.

The truth is, you deserve to be cared for. You deserve to feel safe, loved, and valued. Self-care isn't a luxury—it's a necessity. It's the foundation for creating a healthier, happier life.

So, what exactly is self-care? It's more than just bubble baths and face masks, though those can be enjoyable parts of it. Self-care involves anything that nourishes your mind, body, and spirit. It's about paying attention to your needs and taking steps to address them. It means setting boundaries and saying no when necessary. It's about giving yourself permission to rest, have fun, and simply be.

PRIORITIZING PHYSICAL WELL-BEING

Your body, which has journeyed with you through all experiences, both joyful and painful, holds the echoes of your past.

If your early relationships were inconsistent or filled with fear, your body may have absorbed and carried that emotional turmoil. You might notice tension in your muscles, a racing heart at the slightest hint of conflict, or restless nights as your mind replays anxieties.

These physical symptoms are not separate from your emotional healing journey; they are deeply interconnected. While emotional and mental aspects of healing from disorganized attachment are often emphasized, overlooking the physical component is like trying to solve a puzzle with missing pieces. It's essential to recognize the deep connection between your body and emotions.

Take a moment to pause and listen. Close your eyes, take a deep breath, and tune in to your bodily sensations.

What do you feel? Is there tightness in your chest? A knot in your stomach? A subtle tremor in your hands? These physical signs can provide valuable insights into your emotional state.

Chronic stress and trauma, common in disorganized attachment, can lead to the release of stress hormones like cortisol, which negatively impacts your physical health over time.

Digestive issues, headaches, weakened immune function, and chronic pain can all be linked to the body's stress response. Prioritizing physical well-being is crucial for healing from disorganized attachment.

So, how do we address these physical manifestations? It begins with a commitment to self-care, not as a luxury, but as a necessity.

Self-care isn't just about indulgent activities like bubble baths or face masks (though those can be pleasant), but about intentionally taking care of your body and mind.

Think of self-care as an act of kindness towards yourself, acknowledging that your body deserves attention and care. It's about honoring the vessel that has supported you through so much and rewriting the narrative of neglect and inconsistency that may have been imprinted on your physical self.

Start with the basics: Are you getting enough sleep? Eating nourishing foods that support your body? Moving in ways that feel good? These simple actions can significantly impact your overall well-being.

Additionally, consider activities that specifically address the mind-body connection. Yoga, for example, can help release tension, calm the nervous system, and foster inner peace. Mindfulness practices, such as meditation or focusing on the present moment, can enhance your awareness of bodily sensations and emotions, allowing you to respond with greater compassion and understanding.

NURTURING EMOTIONAL AND MENTAL HEALTH

Emotional well-being involves acknowledging and honoring your feelings, both positive and negative. Allow yourself to experience sadness, anger, or fear without judgment, understanding that these emotions are valid and carry important lessons.

Although you may not have had a safe space for emotional expression in the past, you can create that space for yourself now.

Journaling can be an effective way to release emotions. Writing down your thoughts and feelings helps gain clarity and perspective. If writing seems overwhelming, try alternative forms of expression like drawing, painting, or dancing. The goal is to find healthy outlets that help you process and release built-up emotions.

Mental health, on the other hand, is about maintaining a clear and focused mind. It involves addressing and challenging negative thought patterns that may have developed from early experiences.

Disorganized attachment might leave you feeling unworthy or flawed, but these beliefs are not truths; they are distortions from a time when you were vulnerable and reliant on others.

Cognitive-behavioral therapy (CBT) is a proven method to help identify and reframe negative thoughts. Through practice, you can learn to question and replace these old narratives with more positive and empowering beliefs. Remind yourself that you are worthy, capable, and deserving of love and happiness.

Self-care plays a crucial role in supporting both emotional and mental health. It's not about being selfish; it's essential for your well-being. Self-care can be as simple as taking a warm bath, reading a book, spending time outdoors, or listening to soothing music. Prioritize activities that bring you joy and help recharge your energy.

E X E R C I S E

Create a list of self-care activities that address your physical, emotional, and mental well-being. Make a commitment to engage in at least one self-care activity from each category every week.

Step-by-Step Instructions

Gather Your Materials:

- Materials Needed: Paper and pen or a digital note-taking app.

Create Your Self-Care Categories:

- Action: Divide your paper or digital note into three categories:
  - Physical Well-being
  - Emotional Well-being
  - Mental Well-being

List Activities for Each Category:

- Physical Well-being:
  - Action: Think of activities that help you take care of your body. Write down things like exercise, healthy eating, getting enough sleep, or taking a relaxing bath.

Emotional Well-being:

- Action: Consider activities that nurture your emotional health. Examples might include talking to a friend, journaling, practicing gratitude, or engaging in hobbies you enjoy.

Mental Well-being:

- Action: Identify activities that support your mental clarity and relaxation. This could include meditation, reading, practicing mindfulness, or doing puzzles.

Commit to Your Self-Care Routine:

- Action: Review the list you've created. Choose at least one activity from each category that you can commit to doing every week.
- Weekly Plan: Write down these chosen activities in a weekly planner or calendar, and schedule time for them.

Engage in Your Self-Care Activities:

- Action: Follow through with your self-care plan by engaging in the selected activities each week. Ensure you make time for these activities and enjoy them as a regular part of your routine.

Reflect on Your Experience:

- Action: At the end of each week, take a moment to reflect on how the self-care activities impacted your well-being. Note any changes in your mood, stress levels, or overall satisfaction.
- Questions to Consider:
  - How did these activities make me feel?
  - Did I notice any improvements in my physical, emotional, or mental well-being?
  - Are there any adjustments I need to make to better suit my needs?

Adjust as Needed:

- Action: Based on your reflections, adjust your self-care activities if necessary. Add new activities if you find certain ones are not as effective or if your needs change.

Use the template below for this effect or use it as a guide to create yours.

Physical Well-being

Emotional Well-being

Mental Well-being

Physical Well-being

Emotional Well-being

Mental Well-being

In what areas of my life do I neglect self-care, and why?

____

____

____

____

How can I prioritize self-care to support my healing journey?

____

____

____

____

Chapter 6

TRANSFORMING YOUR INNER NARRATIVE

I remember Lucas well, a client who came to my office in downtown Seattle with a story of profound uncertainty.

His upbringing was marked by the erratic behavior of his mother—sometimes a pillar of support and warmth, other times distant and neglectful.

Our sessions began with Lucas struggling to articulate his feelings of worthlessness. He would often downplay his accomplishments and avoid setting ambitious goals, believing that any success he achieved was merely a fluke. It was clear that his mother's unpredictable care had deeply affected his self-perception. Lucas felt that he was never quite good enough, a belief that had been ingrained in him from a young age.

I suggested we start by focusing on the small victories in Lucas's life. He was hesitant at first, finding it difficult to accept any form of praise or recognition.

To address this, we began with a simple exercise: Lucas would keep a daily log of his achievements, no matter how minor. At first, it was challenging for him to fill even a few lines, but gradually, he began to notice a pattern. Each entry, no matter how small, started to build a new narrative about his abilities and worth.

One particular breakthrough came when Lucas shared a story from his recent promotion at work. He had been given a project to lead, something he initially thought he wasn't capable of handling. To his surprise, the project was a success, and his team had praised his leadership. However, Lucas struggled to internalize this success, attributing it to luck rather than his own skills.

We explored this experience during our sessions, analyzing how his mother's inconsistent caregiving had influenced his ability to accept positive feedback. We worked on reframing these experiences, focusing on evidence of his competence and leadership.

I encouraged Lucas to view this success not as a fluke but as a result of his hard work and skills.

As Lucas began to challenge his negative core beliefs, he also started setting more ambitious goals. He began participating in professional development workshops and took on additional responsibilities at work, something he would have previously avoided.

His newfound confidence was evident not just in his career but also in his personal life. He started to engage more deeply in relationships, setting healthy boundaries and expressing his needs more openly.

Our minds are indeed powerful storytellers, continuously crafting narratives about ourselves, others, and the world. These narratives shape our beliefs, emotions, and actions.

For those who have experienced disorganized attachment, these internal stories can often be fraught with pain and limitation, trapping you in cycles of self-doubt, insecurity, and fear.

However, it's crucial to remember that these stories are not immutable. You have the power to rewrite them and forge a new, more empowering narrative for yourself.

Consider how you speak to yourself when you make a mistake. Do you hear a critical voice berating you, or perhaps a persistent worry about others' judgments? These negative thought patterns can become deeply ingrained, shaping your self-perception and interactions.

They often stem from the unresolved issues linked to disorganized attachment, leaving you feeling unworthy of love and connection, and fostering a sense of isolation and mistrust.

To begin rewriting your internal narrative, start by challenging these negative beliefs. Instead of harsh self-criticism, offer yourself understanding and kindness. Acknowledge that making mistakes is a natural part of being human and that everyone has their own struggles.

Treat yourself with the same compassion you would extend to a friend in a similar situation.

This shift in approach helps dismantle negative self-talk and creates space for a more positive inner dialogue.

Examining and revising your core beliefs is another critical step. Reflect on whether these beliefs are serving you well or holding you back. Are they helping you build the life you aspire to, or are they reinforcing old patterns of insecurity and fear? If your core beliefs are detrimental, it's time to replace them with ones that foster growth and self-acceptance.

This process may be challenging, but it's a vital component of healing and personal development. By rewriting your internal story, you empower yourself to break free from past limitations and embrace a more positive, fulfilling future.

CULTIVATING A POSITIVE SELF-IMAGE

Your self-image plays a crucial role in shaping your life and interactions with others. For those with disorganized attachment, this internal perception might be distorted by self-doubt and past experiences. Yet, with effort and patience, you can clear away these distortions and reveal your true self.

Start by treating yourself with the same kindness and encouragement you'd offer a friend. Recognize and challenge any self-critical thoughts that undermine your confidence. Replace these negative voices with affirmations of your worth and potential.

Shift your focus from perceived shortcomings to what you bring to the table. Embrace your unique strengths, passions, and quirks, understanding that your imperfections are part of what makes you relatable and human.

Celebrate these aspects as they contribute to your individuality.

Engage in activities that help you connect with yourself, whether through creative pursuits like painting or writing, or simply spending time in nature. Such activities can reinforce your self-worth and offer joy.

Accept yourself as you are, acknowledging that self-improvement is a continuous journey. Embrace your progress and celebrate your achievements, no matter how small, to build confidence in your abilities.

As you work on cultivating a positive self-image, you'll find it easier to express yourself, set boundaries, and pursue your goals. This positive self-view will attract relationships and opportunities that align with your true self.

So, take a moment to appreciate yourself, recognizing the masterpiece you are. This journey of self-acceptance and discovery will lead to a more confident and vibrant you.

EXERCISE

Write down your most persistent negative core beliefs. For each belief, challenge it by finding evidence that contradicts it. Replace the negative belief with a more positive and realistic one.

Step 1: Identify Your Persistent Negative Core Beliefs

- Action: Take a few moments to reflect on your most persistent negative thoughts about yourself. These might be beliefs like "I'm not good enough," "I can't trust anyone," or "I always fail."
- Write It Down: List each of these negative beliefs on a piece of paper or in a journal. Try to be as specific as possible with each belief.

Step 2: Challenge Each Negative Belief

- Action: For each negative belief, ask yourself: Is this belief absolutely true? What evidence do I have that contradicts this belief? Look for real-life examples where the belief is not accurate.

Write Contradicting Evidence: Under each negative belief, jot down evidence that contradicts it. For example:

- If your belief is "I always fail," think of times when you've succeeded or overcome challenges, even if they were small victories.

Step 3: Replace the Negative Belief

- Action: Once you've identified evidence against the negative belief, replace it with a more positive and realistic belief. The new belief should be believable and empowering, not overly optimistic. For instance:
  - Old Belief: "I always fail."
  - New Belief: "I sometimes succeed, and I'm capable of learning from my mistakes to improve."

Write the New Belief: Under the contradicting evidence, write your new, more realistic belief that you will consciously choose to adopt moving forward.

Step 4: Reinforce the New Belief

- Action: Practice repeating your new beliefs to yourself regularly, especially in moments of self-doubt or stress. You can also write them down on sticky notes and place them where you'll see them often.

Step 5: Reflect on Your Progress

- Action: After a few days or weeks, revisit your list of new beliefs. Reflect on whether these beliefs are helping you feel more positive and grounded. Adjust them if necessary, based on your experiences.

Example:

- Negative Core Belief: "I'm unlovable."
- Contradicting Evidence: "I have friends and family who care about me and show me love in their own ways."
- New Belief: "I am worthy of love, and I have meaningful relationships that prove this."

Use the templates below for this exercise.

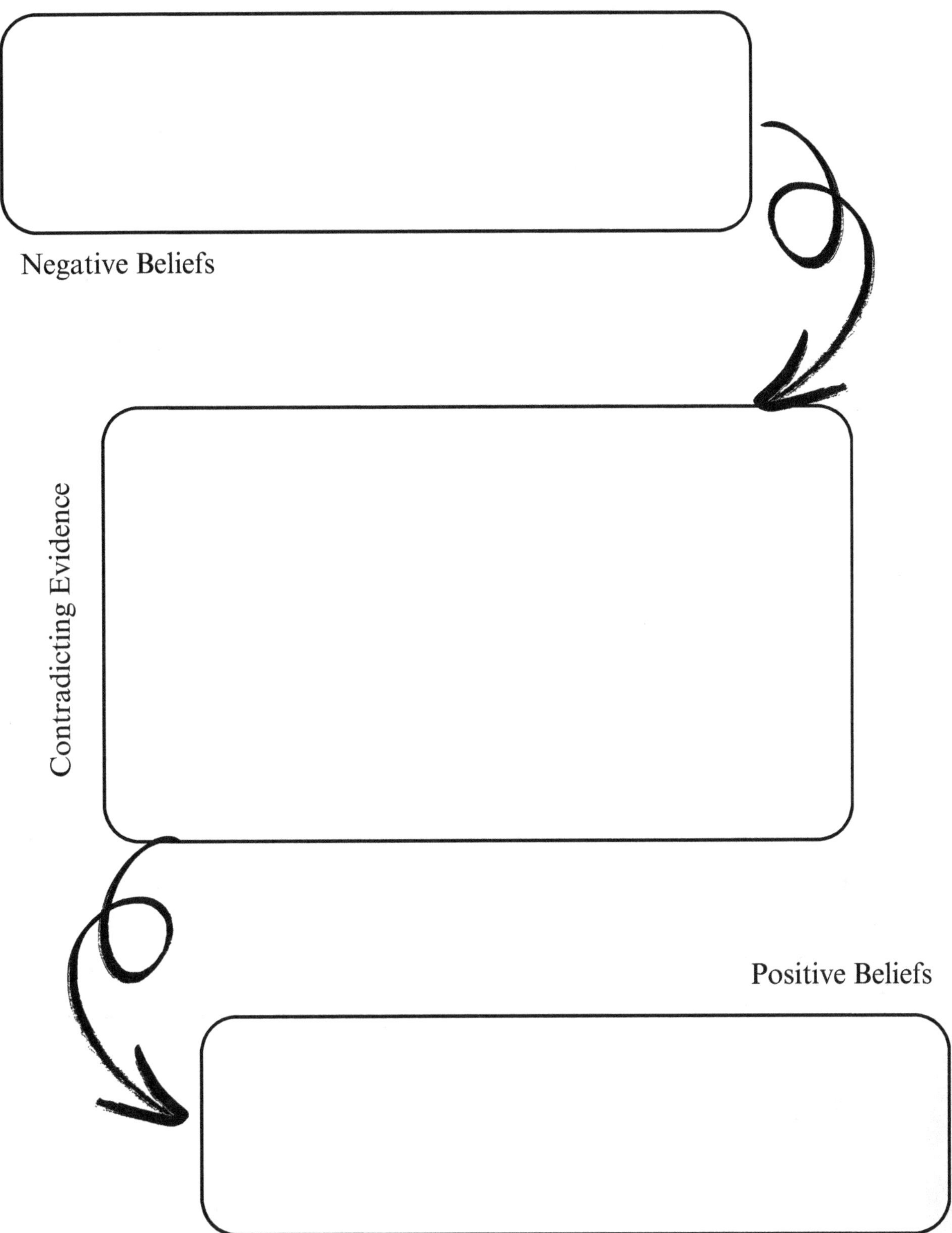

Negative Beliefs
Contradicting Evidence
Positive Beliefs

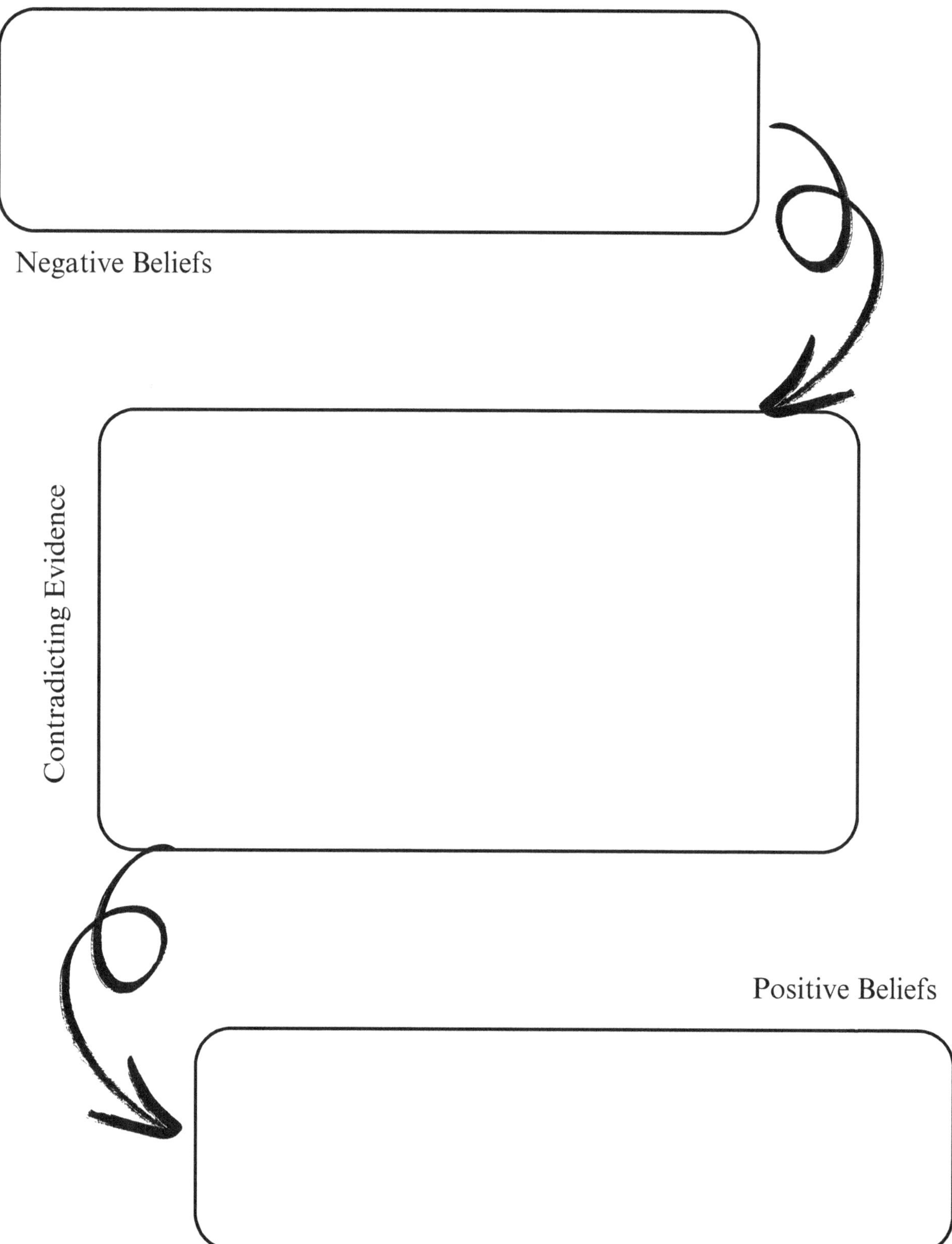

Negative Beliefs
Contradicting Evidence
Positive Beliefs

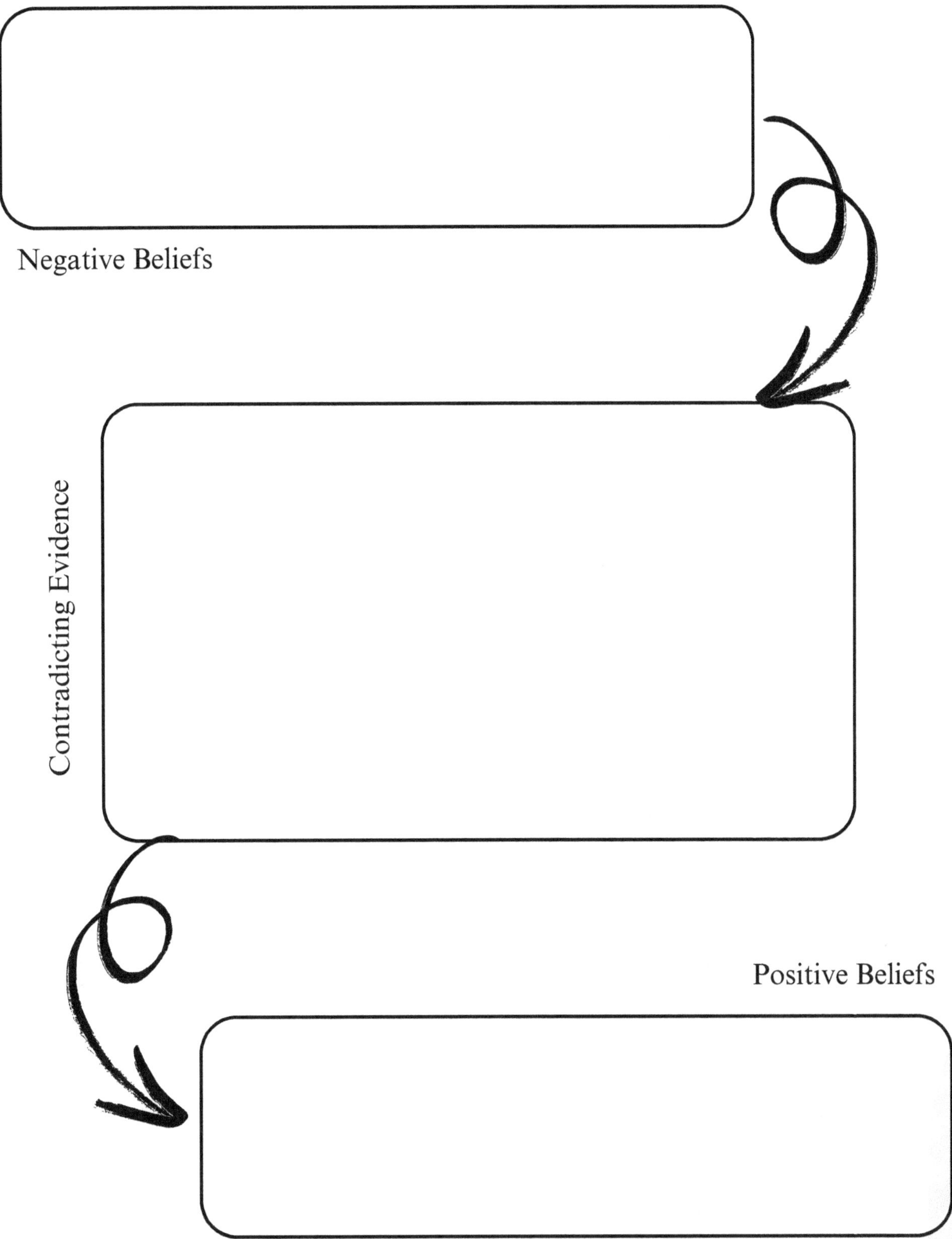
Negative Beliefs
Contradicting Evidence
Positive Beliefs

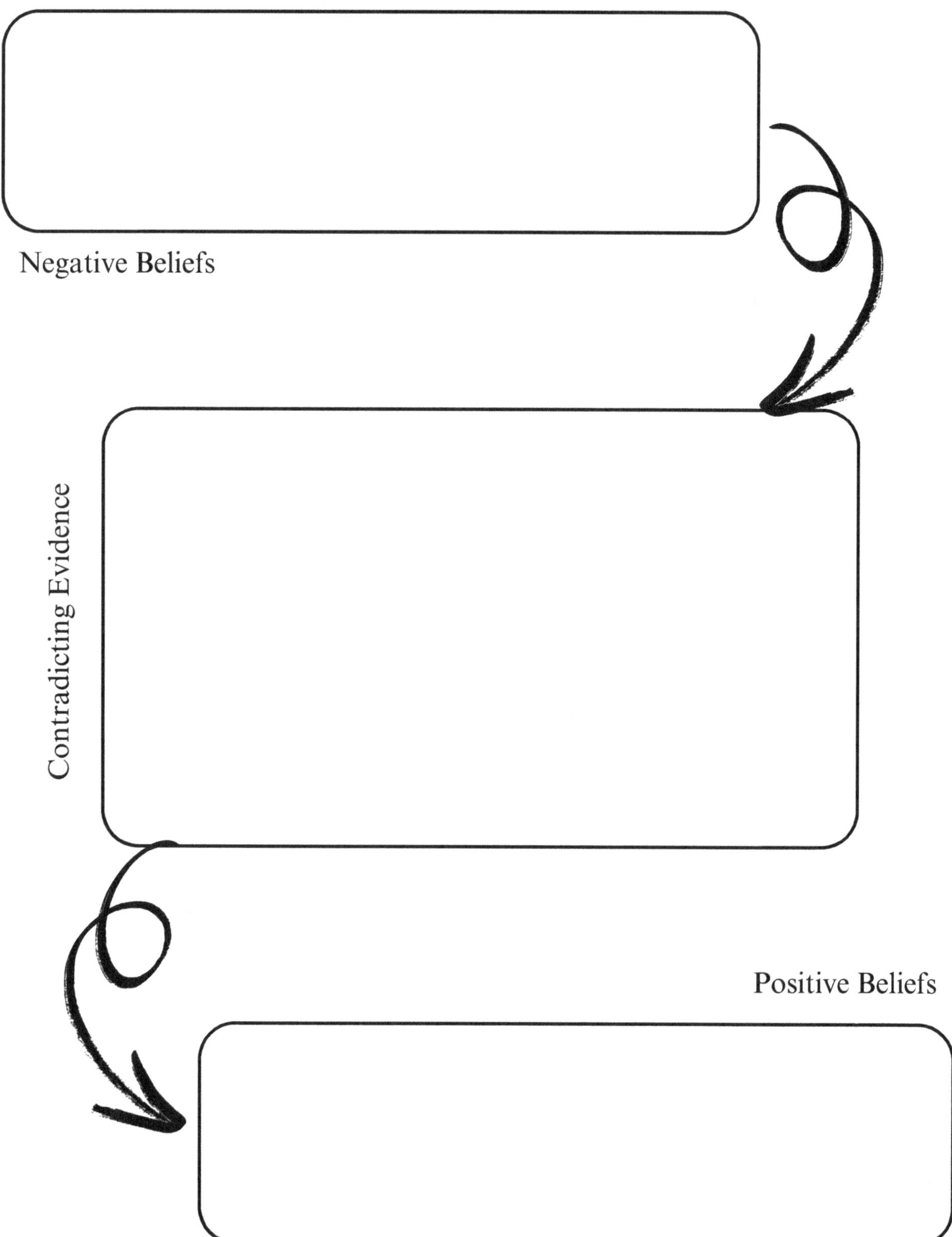
Negative Beliefs
Contradicting Evidence
Positive Beliefs

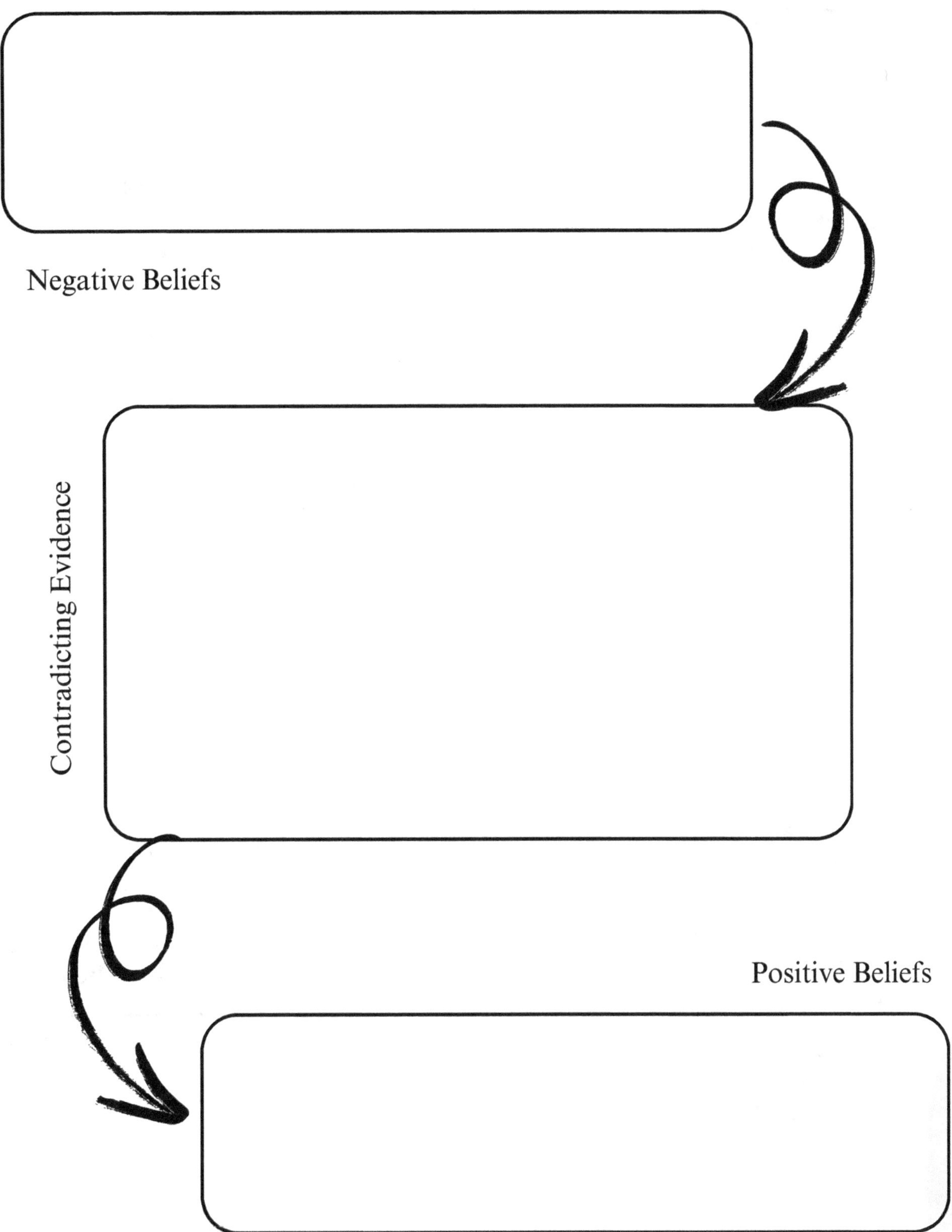

Negative Beliefs
Contradicting Evidence
Positive Beliefs

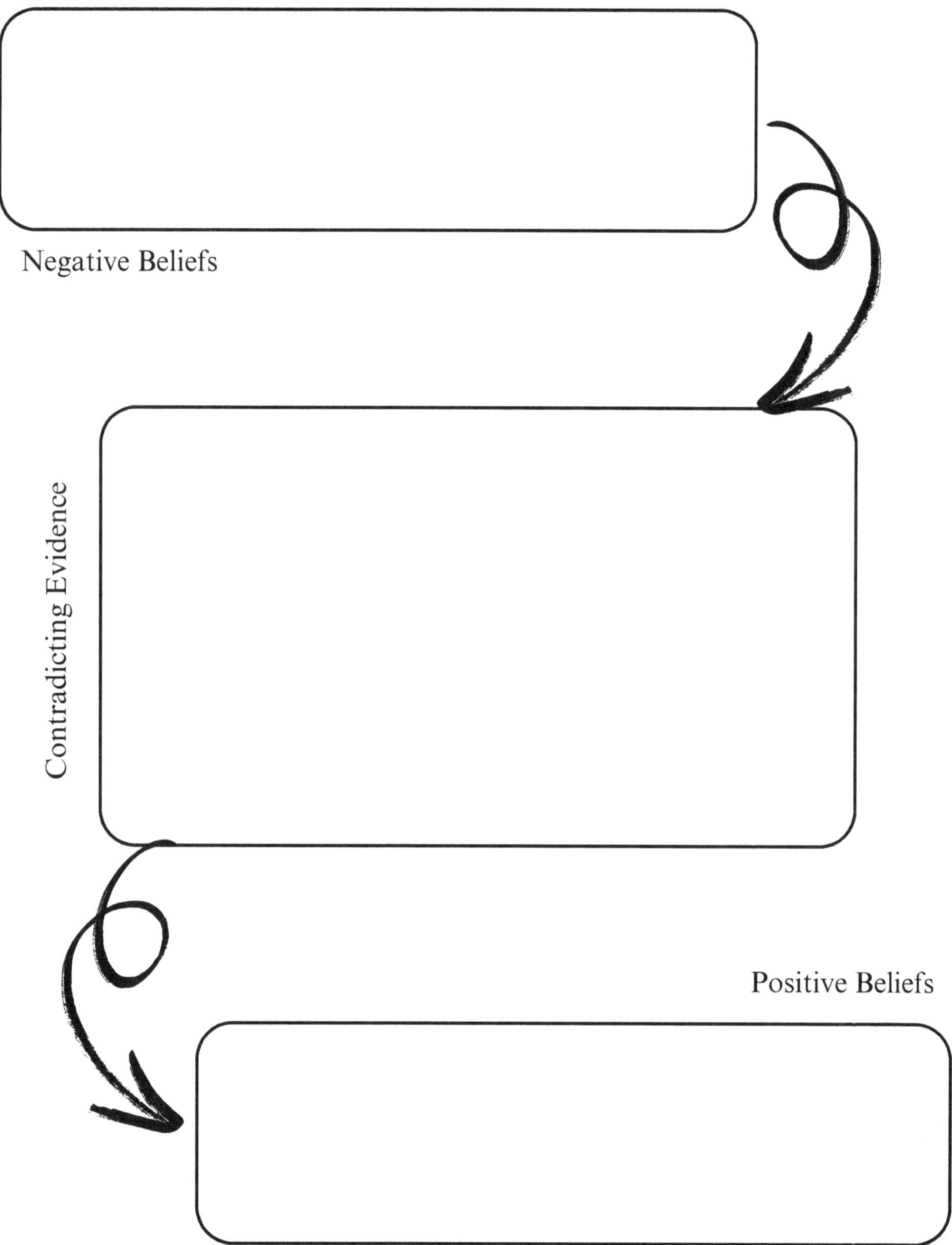

Negative Beliefs
Contradicting Evidence
Positive Beliefs

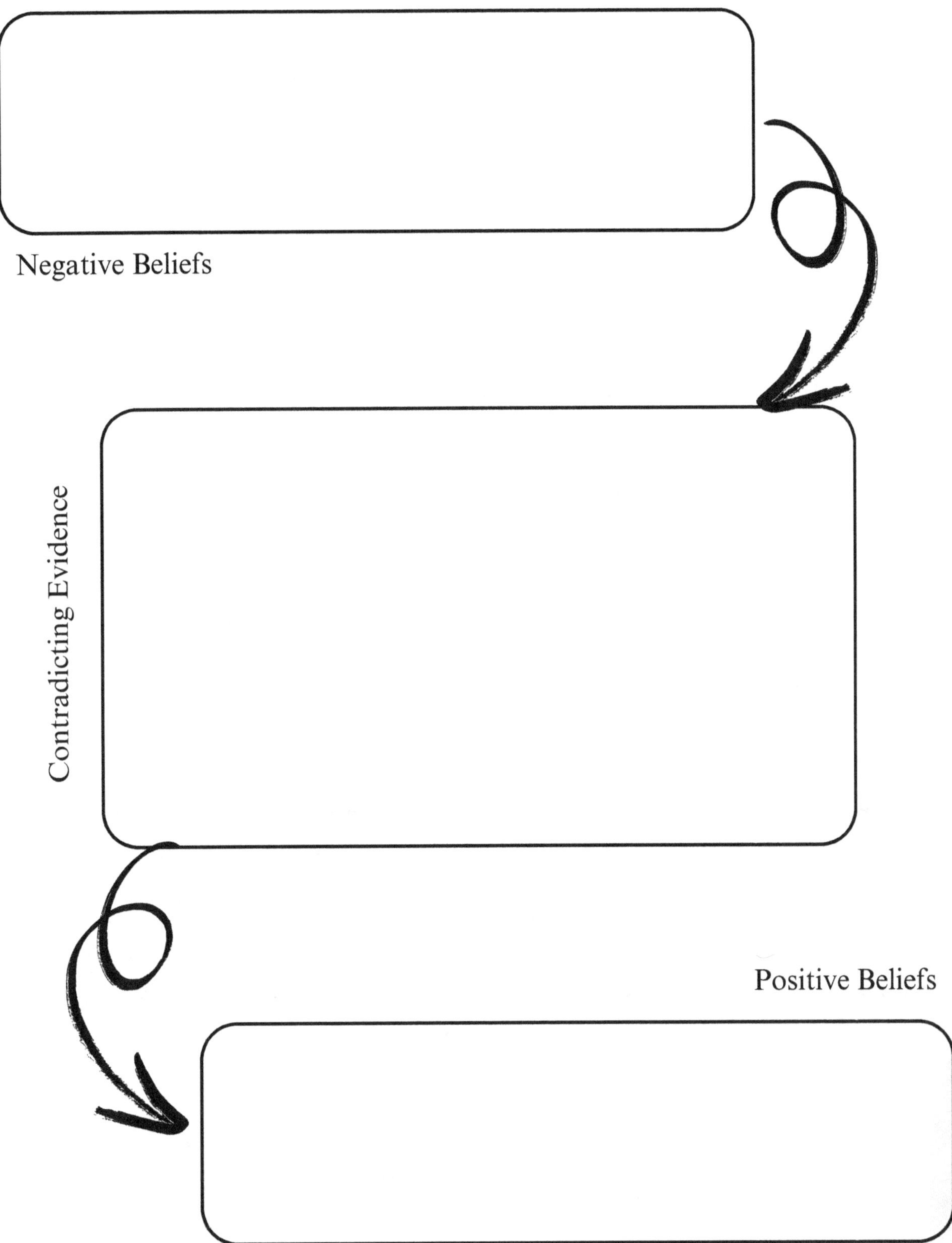

Negative Beliefs
Contradicting Evidence
Positive Beliefs

How do these beliefs affect my self-image and interactions with others?

____

____

____

____

What positive beliefs can I cultivate to transform my inner narrative?

____

____

____

____

Chapter 7

MAINTAINING PROGRESS AND GROWTH

The journey to secure attachment is not a straight line; it's marked by ups and downs, successes and setbacks. Some days, everything feels stable and clear, while on others, doubts cloud your path. Even in these difficult moments, it's essential to remember that the ability to heal, grow, and move forward is always within you.

Research shows that about 15% of the population experiences disorganized attachment, meaning millions of people are dealing with the emotional difficulties associated with it.

The good news is that you're not alone.

Many others have traveled this path, and with the right tools and support, you can reshape your story.

Sustaining progress requires a well-rounded approach. It's about caring for your emotional health, strengthening your relationships, and fostering positive self-talk. It's also about recognizing the triggers that may cause setbacks and developing strategies to cope with them.

A key part of your progress is celebrating even the smallest victories. Whether it's expressing your needs without feeling overwhelmed or reframing negative self-talk with compassion, these are significant milestones on your healing journey.

Building a supportive network is just as crucial. Surround yourself with people who encourage and uplift you, be it friends, family, therapists, or support groups.

These connections provide a safe space to share your feelings and experiences, offering the validation you need.

Continuing to educate yourself on disorganized attachment will also help. The more you understand it, the better you'll be at managing its challenges and fostering secure relationships. Engage in learning through books, workshops, podcasts, and conversations with others who share similar experiences.

Alongside external support, nurturing your inner world is vital. Practice self-compassion and acceptance, reminding yourself that you are deserving of love and connection, despite your struggles. Show yourself the same kindness you would offer a close friend.

Healing from disorganized attachment isn't about perfection. It's about embracing your flaws and understanding that they contribute to your uniqueness. The journey is about making progress, showing up for yourself every day, and continuing to move forward, even when it's tough.

EXERCISE

Draw a map of your support system, including friends, family, and professionals. Identify any gaps in your support network and brainstorm ways to strengthen these connections.

Step-by-Step Instructions:

Gather Your Materials:

- Grab a piece of paper and a pen (or use a digital tool if you prefer).
- Make sure you have some space to write and draw.

Draw the Center Circle:

- Action: In the middle of the paper, draw a circle and write your name inside it.
- Purpose: This represents you, the core of your support system.

Add Circles for Your Support System:

- Action: Around your circle, start drawing other circles for people in your support system. These circles can represent:

- Family members (e.g., parents, siblings, extended family).
- Friends (e.g., close friends, acquaintances, peers).
- Professionals (e.g., therapist, counselor, doctor, mentor, etc.).

- Label: Label each circle with the person's name or their role in your life.
- Proximity: Place circles closer to yours if they are people you rely on frequently, and further away if they're more distant or infrequent sources of support.

Assess Your Support Network:
- Action: Look at your map and reflect on how balanced or complete your support system feels.
- Ask Yourself:
  - Who do I turn to the most for emotional support?
  - Are there areas where I lack support, such as in friendships, family, or professional help?
  - Do I have a variety of support sources, or am I relying too much on one or two people?

Identify Gaps:

- Action: Circle any areas that feel underdeveloped or missing. For example:
- Do I have people who I can talk to when I'm feeling down?
- Is there someone I can go to for advice on specific issues like work, mental health, or personal growth?
- Reflection: Consider what specific types of support might be lacking (e.g., emotional, practical, spiritual).

Brainstorm Ways to Strengthen Your Support System:

- Action: Next to the gaps you identified, jot down ideas for how you could strengthen these connections. For instance:
  - Reconnect with an old friend or make an effort to build new friendships.
  - Reach out to a therapist or join a support group if you need professional guidance.
  - Spend more quality time with family members to deepen your bond.
- Consider: Also think about how you might diversify your support, such as by joining a community group or finding a mentor.

Set Actionable Goals:

- Action: Write down 1-3 specific steps you'll take to improve your support system. These could be:
    - "Schedule weekly coffee dates with a friend."
    - "Research and contact a therapist by next week."
    - "Attend a community event to meet new people."

Review and Update Regularly:

- Action: Periodically revisit your support system map to track changes and progress. As your relationships grow or shift, update the map to reflect new connections and strengthened bonds.

Use the template below or as a guide to complete this exercise.

Support System

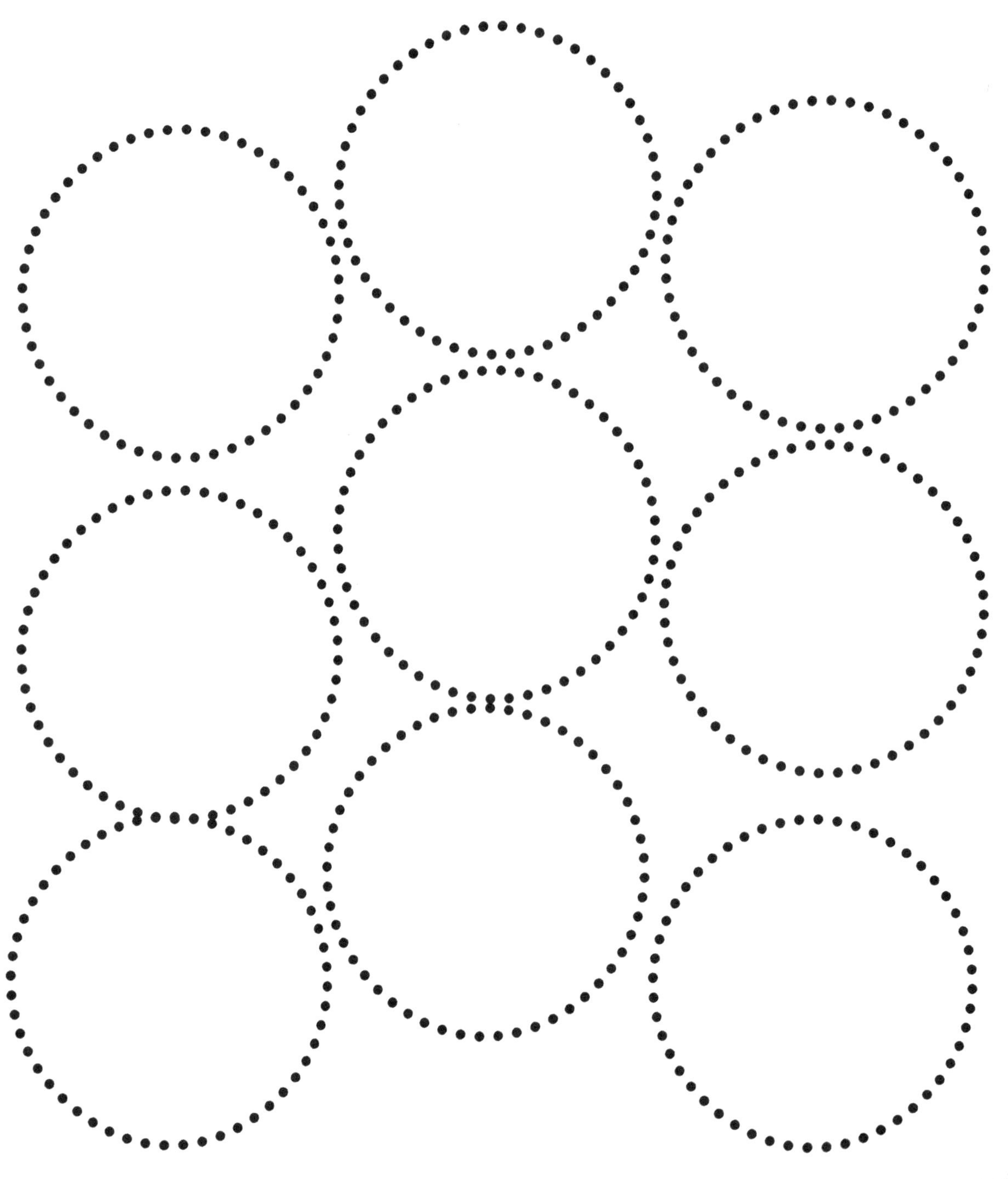

What areas of my support network need strengthening, and how can I address them?

____

____

____

____

Who are the key people in my support system, and how do they contribute to my well-being?

____

____

____

____

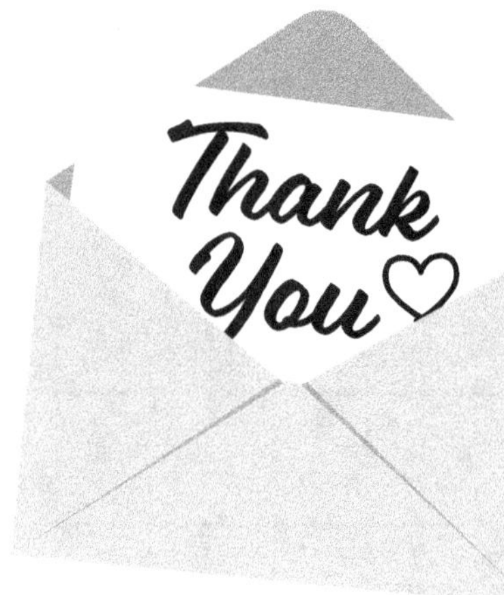

Thank You!

Thank you from the bottom of my heart for taking this journey with me. Your willingness to explore and heal through the "Disorganized Attachment Workbook" means the world.

If you found this book helpful, please consider leaving a review on Amazon—your feedback is invaluable to me and other readers. As a token of my gratitude, scan the QR code for a special bonus gift.

With deepest appreciation,

Isabella Cruz

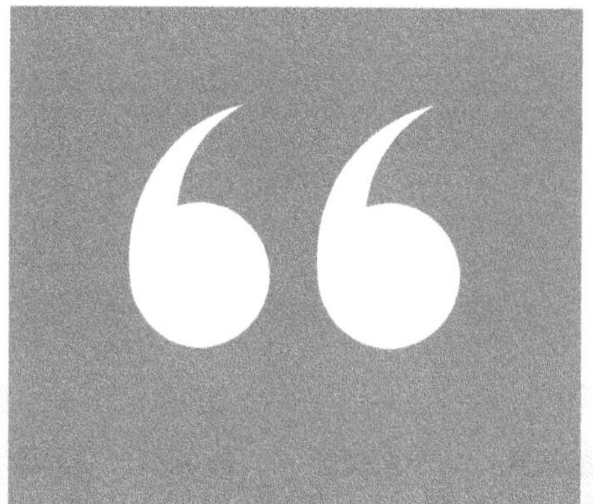

"Love is not about possession. Love is about appreciation." — Osho